stats.con

How we've been fooled by statistics-based research in medicine

James Penston

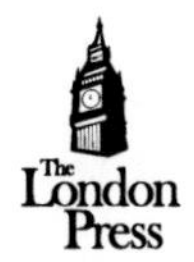

stats.con

ISBN: 978-1-907313-33-2

A Cataloguing-in-Publication (CIP) record for this book is available from the British Library

First published 2010 in the UK by The London Press

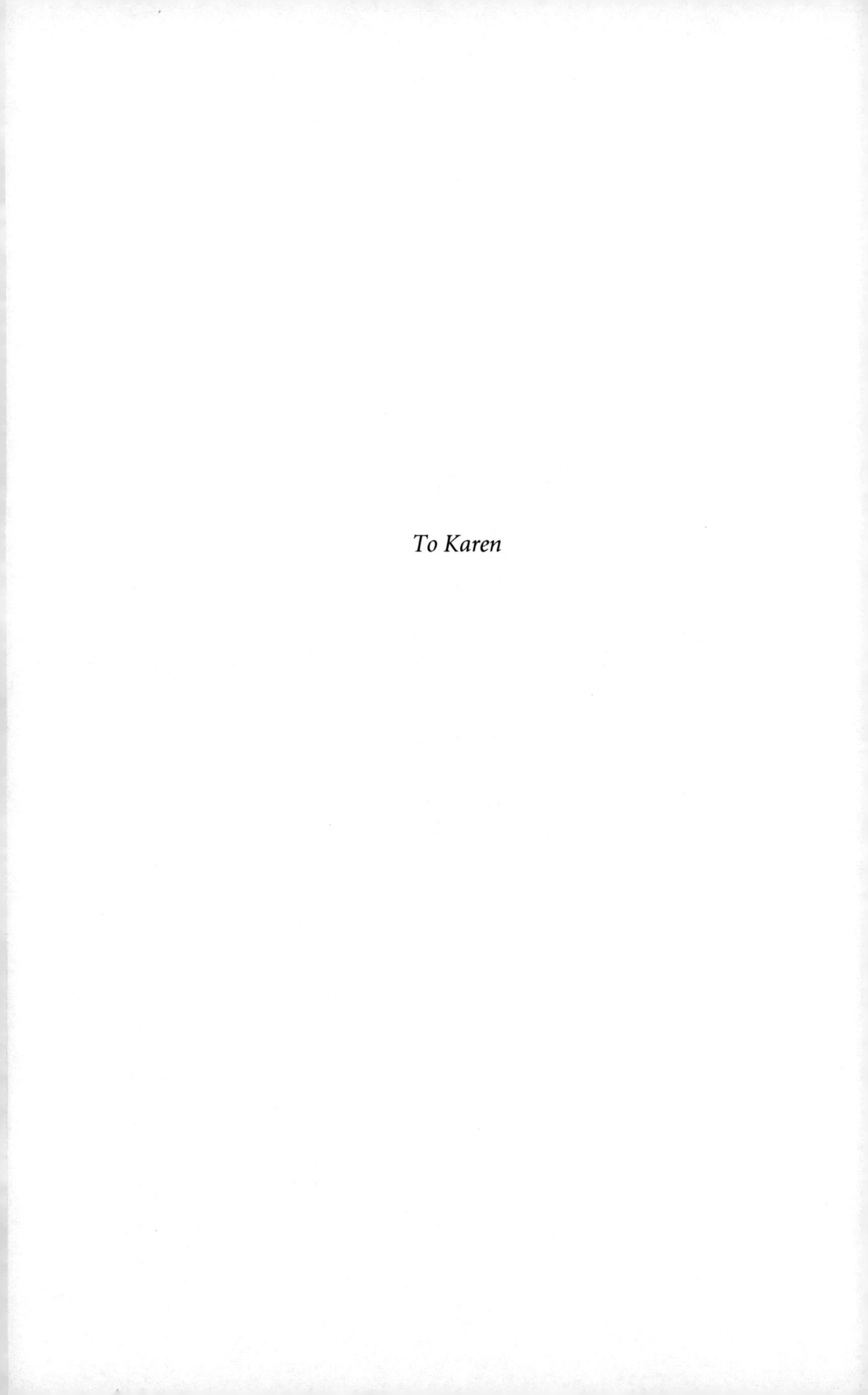

To Karen

Contents

VI. A Squabble of Statisticians 117

Preface

Nowadays, much of what passes for knowledge is derived from statistics-based research. For instance, we're informed that increased government expenditure on schools improves educational standards, that children aren't disadvantaged by being brought up in single-parent families, that speed cameras save lives, that expanding the prison population reduces crime and that passive smoking causes lung cancer. Claims like these are supported by the results of studies involving statistics. This method of research is used widely and affects how we think about education, crime, health, the welfare state, social issues and much else. But how confident should we be about this type of evidence?

Nowhere is the influence of statistics-based research more apparent than in the field of medicine. If the method is flawed, then it has serious consequences for us all. As individuals, the efficacy of many of the treatments we are prescribed is thrown into doubt; as a society, spending vast sums of money on health initiatives may simply be a waste of resources. We need to know whether there is a fundamental problem with statistical studies. But medicine is also the ideal arena in which to explore statistics-based research. More than any other field, it uses the large-scale randomised trial which is generally acknowledged as the most reliable statistical method. If we are to challenge successfully the statistical approach to research, then we must show that this particular type of study is flawed.

We investigate phenomena in the natural world in order to change our surroundings to our advantage – to promote outcomes that are favourable to us and to prevent those that aren't in our interests. In other words, the purpose of research is to identify causal relationships. But can we be sure that statistics-based research achieves this objective?

The aim of this book is to show that causal inference in statistics-based research is unsound and that the product of these studies is of little value. While the arguments focus on medical research, the implications extend far beyond this area into many other academic disciplines that use similar techniques.

This book is intended for medical researchers, practicing clinicians and other health-care professionals, as well as senior NHS managers and academics who formulate health policies. It will challenge their fundamental beliefs and prompt them to question what they currently take for granted. Some, no doubt, will consider the contents of the book to be nothing short of heresy but, hopefully, many more will be persuaded by the arguments and, in consequence, re-think altogether the current fixation with statistics-based research. Patients interested in learning more about the grounds for medical treatments – especially those keen to participate in decisions about their own management – may also find this book valuable. At the very least, they will be better prepared to make informed choices. Finally, those involved in other academic disciplines that use similar methods will recognise the relevance of the criticisms. A successful case against statistics-based research would have repercussions far beyond the field of medicine.

I wish to express my gratitude to Dr Eric Boyd. As a physician with extensive experience in medical research, he is well placed to understand the issues relating to statistical studies. We have spent endless hours discussing these matters over the past decade or more and his advice, as well as his criticism, has been invaluable. But, most of all, his encouragement has been indispensable.

Finally, I would like to thank Dr KG Wormsley. Without him, I would never have had the opportunity to be involved in medical research.

I

The Shadow World of Statistics

It may appear somewhat strange to begin with George Orwell. He wasn't a statistician or a scientist, but one of the most important English literary figures of the 20th century. Yet, despite his lack of any formal training, he had an acute insight into the abuses and dangers of statistics, and the relationship between statistical data and politics.

Again and again, he warned us that statistics are an instrument of the state to control our thoughts and actions. In *Animal Farm*, Squealer used them to persuade the other animals that, contrary to their experience, the revolution had been successful and was delivering an abundance of food.[1] But much worse was to come in *Nineteen Eighty-Four* when statistics, in the hands of Big Brother, became the means of brain-washing the people into falsely believing that, amongst other things, their lives had never been better.

> "Day and night the telescreens bruised your ears with statistics proving that people today had more food, more clothes, better houses, better recreations – that they lived longer, worked shorter hours, were bigger, healthier, stronger, happier, more intelligent, better educated, than the people of fifty years ago. Not a word of it could ever be proved or disproved." [2]

The last sentence of this quotation encapsulates his criticism of statistics. If the data were true, there would be no objection to making them available to the general public. But what if they were false? Orwell painted a picture of the armies of anonymous individuals involved in the collection of large amounts of data and emphasized just how little anyone knew about the process. He described the way in which the figures were manipulated, distorted or even fabricated in order to produce information favourable to those in power. And he repeatedly drew attention to the fact that there was no way of checking the validity of statistics – even personal experiences were unable to contradict them.

The consequences of his analysis are stark. If we don't know how the data are collected, if we can't be sure that they haven't been corrupted and if we have no independent means of verifying them, how can we know whether they are true?

> "And so it was with every class of recorded fact, great or small. Everything faded away into a shadow world in which, finally, even the date of the year had become uncertain." [2]

Orwell, of course, was writing fiction. His arguments aren't technical or presented formally; they are interwoven within his novels. Yet his message is clear: we should view statistics with the utmost scepticism.

We may have avoided the horrors of a totalitarian state, but we haven't escaped the incessant exposure to all kinds of figures designed to influence the way in which we think and act. Our diet of numbers and percentages may be somewhat more refined, but it's there all the same. If we look carefully enough, we'll discover uncertainties with the collection of data, manipulation of the figures and biased interpretation. But most of all, we'll find ourselves in Orwell's shadow-world where truth and falsity are alien concepts.

What the Public Thinks about Statistics

Many people, it seems, view statistics with suspicion. They simply don't believe what they are told. In 2005, the Office of National Statistics published a survey of public opinion regarding a variety of statistics including hospital waiting lists, road traffic accidents, inflation and burglaries.[3] Data were collected from 1,703 individuals by trained interviewers. Approximately one-third of respondents believed that such statistics were generally accurate, one-third held the opposite view whilst the remainder failed to express an opinion. Less than one-fifth of respondents believed that the figures were compiled without political interference and even fewer agreed that the government uses the data honestly when discussing its policies. A clear majority thought that there was political interference and that governments behaved dishonestly when supporting their case with statistics. These findings will come as little surprise to most people.

Survey of Public Opinion about Statistics

	Agree	Disagree	Neither
"Statistics are generally accurate"	37%	31%	32%
"Statistics are produced without political interference"	17%	54%	29%
"Government uses statistics honestly"	14%	60%	26%

Office of National Statistics 2005

The most common reason for the mistrust of statistics – given by almost 60% of respondents – was the belief that the figures may have been manipulated. Others said their personal experience made them question the truth of the figures. Less commonly, respondents suggested that difficulties collecting the data may have contributed to their doubts about the validity.

The idea that an individual's personal experience should be used to question statistical data will have many academics throwing up their arms in horror. It's true to say that a statistical study which reports that speed cameras reduce deaths on the roads isn't falsified by an instance of a fatal accident a few days after the installation of a camera in that same location. But what the advocates of statistics fail to appreciate is that the individual instance is something real, something undeniable, whereas the same cannot be said for the results of a statistical study. Orwell made much the same point in *Nineteen Eighty-Four*. An individual instance may not logically refute a statistical study, but it cannot be dismissed as being irrelevant to the matter.

The ONS survey appears both to reinforce the general impression that statistics are widely mistrusted amongst the general public and to shed some light on the reasons behind these opinions. These data, however, must be interpreted with caution. After all, the findings are themselves statistics. In the present context, it may seem perverse that a statistical study is being used as evidence against statistics. But here we encounter another recurring theme. By their nature, statistical studies are not subject to testing by other methods of investigation. They are simply posited by those who believe in the statistical methods and they stand alone. When the studies produce clear cut and purely descriptive results, as in the case of the ONS survey, we may choose to accept them with the caveat that they may not be accurate. But, too often, the findings are so unimpressive and the conclusions drawn from them so dubious that they are best placed in the wastepaper basket.

Statistics and the State

A sceptical attitude towards statistics is nothing new and may well stem from the close links between statistics and politics. The word *statistics* originates from the Latin *statisticus* – "matters of state" – and subsequently, in the 18th century, from the German *Statistik*, meaning the study of the analysis of government data. By the Victorian times, it had come to refer to numerical information concerning the state and, nowadays, we continue to use the term for data collected by government institutions. We speak, for example, of the "crime statistics", referring to a set of figures each representing the number of offences in various categories committed over a period of one year. And we hear of the latest unemployment rate, the percentage of students passing A-levels, the average length of the waiting lists for operations and the current rate of inflation – all *statistics* to do with government.

By themselves, these statistics have little meaning. They have to be placed in context and this is achieved by presenting them alongside the equivalent data from different times and different locations. Thus, the crime statistics are published together with those of previous years and depicted in graphs or bar charts as trends over time. But this involves something new, something in addition to the presentation of raw statistics. Here, comparisons are being made between the number of crimes at different times and in different places. Inevitably, such comparisons lead to questions concerning these differences. Why is the rate of violent crimes lower in Sweden than in England? What is the cause of the increase in burglary in Scotland over the past five years? If there has been a recent trend, we may, in the absence of any other obvious explanation, conclude that this was due to a particular government policy. But in doing so, we must be sure that there is a real difference – in other words, that the observed difference is not simply due to chance – and that the inference is valid. Here, we encounter a different use of the word *statistics*. In order to make valid inferences and draw conclusions from statistical data, we must adhere to the rules and techniques of the formal discipline known as *statistics*.

Conclusions drawn from statistical data may have serious consequences. This is clearly seen in the sphere of politics. If the latest figures show a steep increase in violent crime, then the government is in trouble; the deterioration will be attributed to current policies and the government's popularity will fall. And a clutch of poor statistics – for example, rising unemployment, increasing numbers of days lost through industrial action and worsening inflation – can spell disaster at the polls as the Labour government found to its cost in 1979.

Politicians

Politicians, however, are fully aware of the dangers and, over many years, they've developed strategies to deal with unwelcome statistics. To begin with, they've acquired a healthy scepticism for numerical data. Perhaps this explains why we are so willing to accept that the most famous quotation related to statistics – "*There are three kinds of lies: lies, damned lies, and statistics*" – was first uttered by Benjamin Disraeli even though its provenance is nowadays disputed.

Politicians have also learned to control statistics. For example, they may alter what is to be collected. During the last Conservative government, the definition of unemployment was changed more than twenty times in an attempt to hide the increasing numbers of people without jobs. In recent times, the classification of various criminal offences, the measures of improvement in the NHS and the criteria for success in education have similarly been tampered with time and again in order to massage uncomfortable figures. Anything that can be done to produce more palatable data will be done. As Winston Churchill cynically remarked,

> "The first lesson that you must learn is, when I call for statistics about the rate of infant mortality, what I want is proof that fewer babies died when I was Prime Minister than when anyone else was Prime Minister. That is a political statistic." [4]

Then, of course, if all else fails, there's always spin. Politicians, ably assisted by their advisors, are experts in the deliberate manipulation of data with the intention of misleading the public. Everyone is aware that the government chooses the days on which to "bury bad news" but it also has another advantage in that official statistics are made available to ministers before the figures are published. As any good politician knows, no data are so easy to manipulate or "spin" as statistics.

Whether on television or radio, in newspapers or in the House of Commons, politicians are adept at handling statistical data. They may not have an inkling about probability theory and few will have ever seen, let alone understood, the complex mathematical formulae, but they know what can and what can't be said about statistical information. In this, they are guided by the words of Lawrence Lowell:

> "... statistics, like veal pies, are good if you know the person that made them, and are sure of the ingredients." [5]

This is all that any street-wise politician needs. The targets are identified. All that remains is to take aim and fire. No wonder politicians are rarely fazed by statistical data. Presented with a study that challenges their position, they simply bring into question the authors or the data. Nowadays, they rarely face the media without being well-briefed. They will be familiar with the reputations, affiliations and vested interests of the researchers. They will also be supplied with a synopsis of the study highlighting its limitations. If required, they can always cherry-pick an alternative study in support of their case, sound in the knowledge that no other research will be able to refute it conclusively.

How many times have we listened to politicians embroiled in an argument bandying statistics with one another? From the *Today* programme on Radio Four to *Newsnight* on BBC1, the format is always the same. The Minister, for instance, believes that children brought up by single parents are disadvantaged whilst the opposition spokesman holds the contrary view. Each resurrects suitably reputable studies in support of their case – the literature, after all, is teeming with contradictory research findings. They vie with each other, casting aspersions on the integrity and independence of the researchers involved in the studies selected by their opponent before picking holes in the data. Wisely, they seldom delve too deeply – they would soon find themselves in uncharted territory. In any case, they want their audience's attention and nothing is more guaranteed to lose it than going into the dry, dusty realms of academic research. Then, of course, there are the inevitable time constraints inherent in programme schedules. When the moment arrives to wrap up the discussion, we're left, as always, with the feeling that it petered out without any winners or losers.

But what if the participants had been experts in sociology? What if there were no time restrictions? What if every relevant study known to man could have been presented and dissected to the point where all of the information available was laid out in the open? It would make no difference. Such is the nature of statistical data that the squabbling would have ended up being as unedifying as that between the politicians. The level of the subject matter and the technical complexity may have been different yet the outcome would have been the same. There is simply too much latitude in the interpretation of statistical studies to allow clear-cut conclusions.

Where there are statistics, there is always room for debate. Nothing is ever settled.

Playing the Statistics Game

Politicians are comfortable with statistics because they know how to play the game. But they're not alone. Many others in public life are equally skilled and only too willing to participate when the occasion demands – from the Chief Constable defending his force's performance in the face of the latest crime figures to the Archbishop arguing that dwindling congregations have nothing to do with the Church's stance on liberal issues.

There is, however, a cost to be paid. The successful player is one who treats statistics with contempt, who seizes on figures favourable to his cause, feigns confidence in them and then attacks his opponent's data knowing full well that his criticisms could just as easily be targeted at his own selection. That pretence and deception are an integral part of the game says much about those who participate in it. But, equally, it exposes the nature of the subject matter. Just as Orwell realised, notions of truth and falsity have no place in the realm of statistics. We may choose to believe that the results of a large study involving many thousands of individual observations permit us to infer something about the natural world but, in so doing, we are merely fooling ourselves. We are playing a game that has lost any contact with reality.

Yet statistics flourish. It's as though we set aside our scepticism and throw ourselves wholeheartedly into the game, as we do when we immerse ourselves in a far-fetched science fiction movie or when we cheer on an athlete despite our awareness of widespread drug-taking in that sport. Of course we don't believe statistics – except, perhaps, when a survey indicates that Germans have the worst sense of humour or that Italian politicians are the most corrupt in Europe.

But not everyone shares this ambivalence. In certain academic circles, the study of statistics is indispensable. Sociologists and psychologists, for instance, depend on statistics for their legitimacy. So, too, do economists and weather forecasters who build statistical models in an attempt to predict the future. Without statistics, their textbooks would comprise mere opinion and they would be banned from referring to their disciplines as a science. Understandably, they defend statistics without reservation for any successful challenge would wipe out their foundations. Unlike politicians, they have to believe in statistics if they are to claim that their subject says anything of importance about phenomena in the natural world.

This brings us to the crux of the matter. In the face of so much scepticism, why is it that sociologists, psychologists, economists and the rest have faith in statistics? How do they know that the results of their studies are valid? How do they know that the inferences they make are legitimate? Bluntly, what is it that they know that we don't?

This book concerns the use of statistics-based research in medicine. Here we see the statistical method in perhaps its most refined form. If it is of value, then it will be shown in this particular case. But if it is proved to be worthless, then the ramifications go beyond medicine to all other disciplines that are grounded in statistics.

References

1. Orwell G. *Animal Farm.* Published by Secker and Warburg, 1945.
2. Orwell G. *Nineteen Eighty-Four.* Published by Martin Secker and Warburg, 1949.
3. ONS Omnibus Survey. Public Confidence in Official Statistics. The Office of National Statistics, March, 2005.
4. Quoted in: Henry Fairlie. The Life of Politics. Methuen, 1968. Pages 203-4.
5. Lowell AL. The Physiology of Politics. The American Political Science Review 1910;4;1-15.

II

Crooked Thinking

Perhaps it was the appearance in the *British Medical Journal* of the first published randomised controlled trial in 1948.[1] Or maybe it was Doll and Hill's epidemiological study of the relationship between smoking and lung cancer in 1950.[2] Whatever the precise event, we may say that sometime, shortly after the end of the Second World War, medical research fell under the spell of statistics. For the most part, it went unnoticed. There was no fanfare, no fuss. But this belied its importance. It was nothing short of a revolution in thinking that was to change the way research was carried out and, in time, that would affect the lives of countless millions of people around the world.

The alliance between medicine and statistics was anticipated to lead to untold benefits. There was the promise of solutions to the seemingly intractable problems that hampered the search for the causes of disease and thwarted efforts to discover effective treatments. Few, though, were aware that they were taking the first tentative steps along a slippery slope that would lead to the woeful state of affairs that is much of today's medical research.

The Problems Facing Medical Researchers

By the middle of the 20th century, it had become clear that a new approach to establishing the causes of disease was required. For fifty years or more, the Henle-Koch postulates[3] had dominated the investigation of causation in medicine – indeed, they are still referred to in textbooks and journals today. It is, though, worth remembering that they were formulated in an era rich in discoveries in bacteriology. In the space of just a few decades, *Bacillus anthracis, Mycobacterium tuberculosis, Vibrio cholerae, Salmonella typhi, Mycobacterium leprae* and *Corynebacterium diphtheriae* had been identified as the causes of anthrax, tuberculosis, cholera, typhoid, leprosy and diphtheria, to name but a few. It was, therefore, only to be expected that Jacob Henle's original postulates, modified by his pupil Robert Koch, focussed on the identification of causal relationships between bacteria and disease. For example, two of the postulates stipulated that the organism must be present in every case of the disease and that it must be capable of producing the disease in healthy recipients. Thus, the fundamental idea behind the Henle-Koch postulates was that a cause is both necessary and sufficient for the occurrence of the disease.

But this interpretation of causation rests uneasily within medicine. Tissues and organs have only limited ways of responding to injury and there are no grounds for believing that a particular pathological lesion has only one cause. There are, for example, many different bacteria – as well as other infective agents including viruses, fungi and protozoa – that may produce pneumonia. Hence, we can't say that *Streptococcus pneumoniae,* the organism most commonly associated with pneumonia, is a necessary cause of this illness. Neither can we say that a particular organism is a sufficient cause for the disease. There are many different factors which affect whether or not exposure to an organism will produce a disease, not least innate or acquired immunity. Moreover, there are practical difficulties with the identification of infective agents that limit the application of the Henle-Koch postulates, including the reliability of tests to isolate the organism and the availability of susceptible animal hosts in which to demonstrate that the disease occurs after exposure.

Thus, even in the context of bacterial disease, the Henle-Koch postulates were, from their inception, too restrictive for the identification of cause and effect relationships. Then, advances in medicine in the first half of the 20th century added further weight to the calls for an alternative approach to disease causation. The discovery of viruses posed particular problems. The bacteriological model – with its emphasis on culture of the organism and transmission of the disease – was no longer suitable. Viral illness was diagnosed on the basis on serological testing for antibodies rather than isolation of the causative agent, while culture and methods to show transmission were not routinely available. But it was developments in chronic diseases that, perhaps, most threatened the Henle-Koch postulates. It became recognised that many diseases were multi-factorial – in other words, the presence of the disease depended on a number of different causal factors – and, therefore, it was no longer possible to think in terms of necessary or sufficient causes. And, of course, most chronic diseases in developed countries are not the result of bacteria, or, for that matter, other infectious agents. The Henle-Koch postulates had passed their sell-by date.

At about the same time, clinical researchers were facing a different problem. In the pre-antibiotic era, the mortality from lobar pneumonia due to *Streptococcus pneumoniae* was approximately 33% depending on a number of factors many of which were unknown. This variation in outcome made assessment of the efficacy of treatment difficult. Consider, for example, a group of patients with pneumonia who all survive after being treated with antibiotics. It would clearly be wrong to conclude that this demonstrated the effectiveness of the medication – the group might have been made up of patients with a particularly favourable outcome regardless of treatment. The solution to this problem, of course, is to use controls. The theory is straightforward: two groups of patients are matched as closely as possible for factors related to the outcome and only one group is given the active treatment; if the only difference between the groups is the presence or absence of treatment, then any difference in outcome may be attributed to treatment. But the simplicity of this approach hides the practical difficulties of selecting two groups of patients equally matched in terms of all relevant factors, both known and unknown. Despite many attempts to devise ways of producing equal groups, no convincing method emerged. It always remained possible to attribute any difference in outcome to factors other than the treatment. This was the problem that continued to bedevil clinical researchers throughout the first half of the 20th century.

The Promise of Solutions

In an important way, the two problems – the identification of the cause of disease and the demonstration of the efficacy of treatment – are similar. In both cases, it's a matter of the legitimacy of causal inference. And, in each case, statistics claimed to have the answer.

With regard to disease causation, the solution proposed was that of carefully controlled epidemiological studies. For example, a group of individuals exposed to the cause were to be compared with a control group, selected to be as similar as possible in all known characteristics but with no history of exposure. If the proportion of individuals developing the disease was greater in the exposed group, then – provided certain conditions were satisfied, including the demonstration that the difference was statistically significant – a causal relationship was said to have been established.

Statistics in Medical Research

	Disease Causation	Clinical Trials
Problem	Failure of Henle-Koch postulates Diseases with multiple causes	Ensuring observed difference between groups is due only to treatment effect
Solutions	Statistical approach to causation Epidemiological studies	Randomised controlled trials Statistical analysis

When it came to testing new treatments, there was even more on offer. RA Fisher's seminal work [4] on randomised experiments in the 1920's caught the imagination of medical researchers and, in due course, led to the first randomised controlled clinical trial in 1948. By randomising patients to the different treatment groups, all relevant factors would be distributed equally amongst the groups and, thus, any difference in outcome could be reliably attributed to the treatment. Not only that, but randomisation provided a sound basis for the use of statistical tests.

On the surface, it may seem that epidemiological studies and randomised controlled trials have little in common. This is certainly true when it comes to the selection of controls and use of deliberate intervention. Yet, they share a fundamental feature: in each case, a situation is created in which the observed difference between the groups – provided that it is statistically significant – is claimed to justify causal inference. As we will see, though, this turns out to be a major flaw in statistics-based research.

The Triumph of Statistics

Within just a few generations, the statistical approach has come to dominate much of research and, in turn, the practice of medicine.

Now, undergraduates, from the moment they enter medical school, are exposed to epidemiological studies and randomised trials. They attend courses in statistics and have to demonstrate an understanding if they are to pass examinations. Postgraduate education, too, reinforces the statistical approach and proficiency is required for progress in most careers in medicine.

When it comes to medical research, it's nowadays considered mandatory that statisticians be involved in the design, analysis and interpretation of the results of epidemiological studies and clinical trials. In effect, little may be done without their agreement and participation. And the consequence is, of course, that research departments – whether in academia or in the pharmaceutical industry – are teeming with statisticians. The editors of medical journals, too, have encouraged the proliferation of both statistics and the exponents of that trade. They demand statistical analysis in all published research studies and increasingly use statisticians for peer review of submitted manuscripts.

However, the best evidence of the extent to which statistics have conquered medical research is to be found in the publications from the Royal Colleges and the National Institute for Health and Clinical Excellence (NICE). Open any of the clinical guidelines and, within a few paragraphs, you'll be greeted with the ritual exposition of the "hierarchy of evidence". In pride of place, you'll find randomised controlled trials and their offspring, meta-analyses. These are the most trusted and revered of all research methodologies. In second place are the epidemiological studies which, although not quite meeting the exalted standards of RCTs, still command respect from the medical community. But as for the rest… it's almost as if they don't count. All other work is relegated to the realms of uncontrolled data, opinion and hearsay – as such, they're considered to be next to worthless.

Thus, the only studies that are believed to be valuable are those based on the statistical approach. This is the basic tenet of the religion known as Evidence-Based Medicine. A claim supported by large-scale randomised trials or epidemiological studies will be accepted without question; one based on thirty or forty years of clinical experience will be derided as being anecdotal. The blinkered world-view of the EBM zealots has profoundly changed the nature of medicine. Doctors are now challenged for not acting in line with EBM. They are under the control of NICE, the Royal Colleges and government diktat. Their professional freedom is now so severely restricted that their role in medicine is under threat. Such is the triumph of statistics.

A Hollow Victory

The statistical approach to medical research, therefore, has triumphed. But this is true only in terms of its influence and the way it's been adopted all around the world. It's reflected more in the acceptance of an idea – in other words, that of a particular research methodology – than success in delivering major advances in medicine. Epidemiological studies haven't been responsible for the discovery of the causes of many diseases, nor have large randomised trials produced many drugs that have materially altered the lives of patients. The promises have proved to be empty.

Any impartial judge would find it hard to conclude that statistics-based medical research is anything other than a failure. That it has flourished is due to the presentational skills of its advocates and the lengths to which they will go in order to persuade us of the correctness of their views.

Product promotion

Today, it seems that almost any product may be sold successfully. We only have to think of the enormous sales of bottled water, vitamin pills and anti-ageing creams. It's simply a question of marketing. A product may be beneficial, may make no difference or may actually do us harm. But it doesn't matter. As long as the marketing strategy is correct, many of us will buy it. This applies as much to ideas as it does to material things. Political manifestos and religions are prime examples. So, too, is the statistical approach to research.

What began with the conversion of relatively few influential figures became, within a couple of decades, a widely accepted belief. The speed with which the idea spread is certainly impressive. In the early years, this was driven by the promise of solutions to the difficulties facing medical research. But there were other factors. The importance of having the support of medical journals can't be overstated. They've constantly reinforced the superiority of studies based on statistical methods and compelled researchers to comply or face rejection of their work. Medical schools have also played their part by introducing the statistical approach to research into the curriculum.

More recently, the promotional campaign on behalf of statistics-based research – typified by the ubiquitous hierarchy of evidence – has paid dividends. The randomised trial is now accepted to be the "gold-standard". Regulatory authorities have further entrenched statistics into research. Then, of course, there was the birth of the EBM movement with its devotion to all things statistical.

There's something about the hierarchy of evidence that smacks of religion. The way in which it appears at the start of each set of guidelines serves as a reminder to readers of the basic tenets of their faith and creates the correct frame of mind to interpret the substance of the document. There's an air of dogma; there's no room for doubt. The hierarchy is simply posited as the truth, as if it were copied from the Holy Scriptures. Nonetheless, it's an effective marketing ploy. If something is said often enough, people will believe it and the incessant reiteration of the hierarchy has ensured headline exposure for the statistical approach. And what makes it all the more effective is that the message comes from those in authority. Shameless brain-washing it may be, but it works.

As a marketing exercise, the conversion of the entire medical profession to statistics-based research has been a remarkable success. Not that medicine is the only discipline to have embraced that methodology. We've already noted that psychology and the social sciences have succumbed to an equal, if not greater, degree and many others have followed in their wake.

Protecting the product against attack

But no matter how skilful the marketing, more has been needed. Measures have had to be taken to hide the problems associated with statistics-based research. Here, the advocates have been only too willing to defend their product by fair means or foul.

Hiding the flaws

Obfuscation has been a prime weapon in this defence. With the passage of time, weaknesses and faults in research have been detected and, as each problem surfaces, alterations have been made. Frequently, though, the changes either expose further defects or create new ones. As a consequence, epidemiological studies and large RCTs have evolved into complex structures. The published papers are long and detailed, involving highly technical aspects that make them impenetrable to all but the most well-informed. Numerous errors may occur that threaten the integrity of the findings yet these are far from easy to detect. Indeed, the information provided in the publication is often ambiguous, incomplete or missing altogether, thus preventing even those who are conversant with the methodology from accurately appraising the work. In general, most doctors and nearly all lay people would find such publications inaccessible and, hence, even if they had the time and the inclination to read them carefully, they would be unlikely to detect anything amiss.

Manipulation of data

Selective reporting and data manipulation to make the results more favourable appear to be standard practice. The dark arts of spin, it seems, are as much a part of medical research as they are of politics. Exaggerated or misleading claims are commonplace and frankly untrue statements are not unusual.

For example, results are commonly presented in terms of relative risk, rather than the more meaningful and accurate absolute risk. This is a practice that is well recognised to persuade the unwary that the results of a study are evidence of a major advance when, in fact, this is untrue. But, while such manipulation may be seen as solely the work of individual researchers to promote their particular studies, it plays a more general role. Lowering the thresholds for the definition of success in epidemiological studies and clinical trials creates the illusion that medical research based on statistics delivers more valuable results than is actually the case.

Re-writing history

It's entirely predictable that the proponents of statistics-based research are keen to re-write the history of medicine. By exaggerating the failures and playing down the successes of the past, they encourage a more favourable judgment on modern research.

Such is the hegemony of statistics that anyone reading textbooks and journals would be forgiven for believing that, before the middle of the 20th century, medical research was languishing in the dark ages when nothing of any value was produced. After all, the towering figures of earlier times weren't familiar with the concepts of P-values, confidence intervals, t-tests and analysis of variance. Yet there had been great advances in medicine long before the statisticians assumed centre stage. Enormous strides had been taken in physiology, biochemistry and pharmacology. So, too, in microbiology where, by the end of the 19th century, the causative organisms for many diseases had been identified followed, within a few generations, by the discovery of antibiotics used to treat previously lethal infections. Surgeons operated successfully – on the heart and lungs, the gastrointestinal tract, the kidneys and bladder, the uterus and ovaries, endocrine glands, bones, skin, eyes, and nervous system – with the assistance of effective anaesthetics and muscle relaxants. And all without a statistician in sight.

But the advocates of the statistical approach conveniently choose to ignore the earlier successes. They focus instead on the errors of the past. With tedious repetition, their writings resurrect blood letting as the cardinal example of what was wrong with medical research before it was rescued by statistics. They mock their forebears as inept quacks whose practice harmed more patients than it cured. But they should be wary. At least the physicians of the past didn't spend their time rounding up millions of healthy individuals and applying dubious illness labels to them before commencing long-term drug treatment based on the most flimsy of data. Future generations may reasonably judge that the EBM zealots with their obsession with statistics have caused more harm than their predecessors who at least targeted their treatments to patients with disease.

Crooked Thinking

The statistical approach was originally introduced in the context of small randomised trials. For example, the now famous 1948 MRC trial of streptomycin in pulmonary tuberculosis involved only 107 patients.[1] It's of some interest that, during the celebrations of the fiftieth anniversary of the first published RCT, Doll remarked that it had been considered necessary to introduce the new methodology gradually, using small numbers of patients, in order to promote its acceptance.[5] This was certainly a shrewd move. It's relatively easy to argue the case for randomisation and statistical analysis in small studies but, as Doll hinted, it was a different matter persuading the medical community in the early years that large-scale studies associated with small treatment effects were worthwhile. Such a move had to wait until the general principle of randomised trials had been accepted widely. It was only after a period of indoctrination that the more extreme version of the statistical approach came to the fore. It took several decades and, even then, it had to be brought in by stealth. Over time, larger and larger clinical trials appeared in the literature, each year surpassing the previous record, while the size of epidemiological studies increased in parallel with that of RCTs. Nowadays, journals regularly publish studies involving tens of thousands of participants and still there are calls for even larger numbers to be recruited in the future. Barely an eyebrow is raised. The deception conjured up more than fifty years ago worked exactly as planned.

But why did the early advocates of statistics bother so much about concealing their intentions? Presumably, they believed in what they were doing. Perhaps they feared that others wouldn't understand and, consequently, that the entire project might be ruined. But, even according to this charitable account of their behaviour, they were guilty of crooked thinking. Somehow, though, subsequent generations failed to notice and the crooked thinking survives to this day.

Size matters. It matters in everyday life. Whether we're thinking of buildings, sports stadiums, cars, planes, televisions or freezers, we prefer them large. We want the weightiest beef-burgers and the deepest buckets of fried chicken, while wine must be served in a half-pint schooner and coffee in a small barrel. Big is beautiful. And what's true of life in general is true also of medical research. The bigger the study, the better it must be. Researchers in their publications boast about the many thousands of patients recruited, pharmaceutical companies in their promotional materials brag about the enormous size of the study sample, while advocates of the statistical approach nod approvingly before asking for even more. Quite simply, it's taken as axiomatic that these mega-trials are, by virtue of their size, of the utmost value. But the truth is that the huge numbers do not reflect strength but weakness.

Large trials are required because the expected therapeutic benefit is so small and this, in turn, is a function of ignorance. For example, because researchers lack sufficient knowledge to identify which patients with hypertension would develop a stroke, they recruit a large, heterogeneous sample of which only a small proportion would suffer from that outcome in the absence of any treatment. And researchers also have an inadequate understanding of the mechanism of the drug treatment which leads to a situation in which only a minority of those patients who would have developed a stroke actually benefit from treatment. Thus, the difference in outcome between treatment and placebo is very small indeed and, if this is to be shown to be statistically significant, large numbers of patients have to be recruited.

The Inverse Law of Study Size

The size of the study is inversely proportional to...

- Knowledge of the subject matter
- The size of the treatment effect
- The value of the results to individual patients
- The overall importance of the study

The large size of a study isn't chosen because it's intrinsically valuable – on the contrary, it's a reflection of the limitations of knowledge concerning the subject matter. But how often do we see this out in the open? It's concealed because it throws into doubt the value of large-scale statistical research. How many doctors who treat patients directly on the basis of the results of statistical studies really appreciate the significance of the size? The answer, of course, is very few. And this is precisely what those in the EBM movement want because it allows them to claim important successes where none actually exist.

Conclusions

In the mid-20th century, medical researchers weren't alone in finding the allure of statistics irresistible. It was very much a feature of the times and other academic disciplines, notably psychology and the social sciences, followed the same path.

Statistics promised much but has subsequently delivered little. Yet, due to the allegiance of its followers, the flaws and failings have, for the most part, remained hidden. The promotion of the statistical method has been extremely effective. Judged by its widespread adoption and pervasive influence, statistics has triumphed. But it's a victory of presentation over substance. What has held the enterprise together has been the willingness of the advocates of statistics-based medical research to adopt any measures necessary to ensure success as well as the gullibility of everyone else to accept without question what they are told.

The statistical approach is touted as a major advance in medical research and, to all intents and purposes, continues unchallenged. It's truly astonishing that the authors of published papers, the sponsors of the studies, the editorial writers and the lay press, together with all those who quote the studies, whether verbally or in print, can speak approvingly of the large size of the study without fear of ridicule. Large studies should be mentioned in hushed tones with an air of contrition for they tell a tale not of strength but of weakness.

But this is only scratching the surface. The crooked thinking associated with the statistical approach to medical research, as we shall see, goes much deeper.

References

1. Medical Research Council. Streptomycin treatment of pulmonary tuberculosis. BMJ 1948;ii;769-82.
2. Doll R, Hill AB. BMJ 1950;ii;739.
3. Koch R. Ueber bakteriologische Forschung. In: verh X. Int Med Congr Berlin 1890. Page 35; 1892.
4. Fisher RA. Statistical methods for research workers. 1925.
5. Doll R. Controlled trials: the 1948 watershed. BMJ 1998;317;1217-20.

III

Epidemiology – The Study of Scare Stories

Introduction

As judged by the number of published studies in recent times, epidemiology is flourishing and this is confirmed by the position given to this type of research in the hierarchy of evidence.

Over the years, epidemiology has had notable successes. The demonstration of a causal link between smoking and lung cancer by Doll and Hill in the 1950's was, without doubt, an important advance in medicine.[1] But the high esteem in which epidemiology is held rests on past glories. Nowadays, it produces little of real value.

The emphasis on statistics in medical research has led directly to the acceptance of studies reporting small effects. Statistical significance has become the yardstick by which research is judged and the size of the P-value, rather than the magnitude of the effect, is now the arbiter of what is considered worthwhile. This is as true of epidemiological studies as it is of clinical trials. But small effects are seldom important. What's more, they're a poor guide to the presence of cause and effect relationships. Inevitably, this has led to a profusion of unwarranted claims of benefit and harm. What we eat and drink, where we live, how we travel, our habits and pastimes – every aspect of our lives has, at one time or another, been brought into question by the finding of small effects in epidemiological studies. But the research often delivers inconsistent findings. A familiar pattern emerges: one day, red wine is condemned, the next, it's said to protect us against heart disease... one day, coffee causes cancer, the next, it doesn't... and so on. The general public are rightly beginning to view the results of epidemiological research with suspicion and even ridicule.

Epidemiological Studies and Causal Inference

Epidemiological studies are usually classified into two main groups, namely, descriptive and analytic. Typically, descriptive studies collect data and report on the distribution of certain characteristics within the sample under investigation. For example, cross-sectional studies or surveys in medicine may describe the prevalence of diseases like rheumatoid arthritis or multiple sclerosis in the general population. Data may be collected at different points in time allowing a description of the trends in a disease as, for instance, in the case of the annual mortality from lung cancer. Cohorts of individuals may be followed over long periods of time to determine the incidence of various diseases or to describe the natural history of a disease. The essential point about these studies is that, although they provide useful information, they don't involve a control group and, therefore, preclude causal inference. Descriptive studies, however, may offer clues about possible causes and prompt further investigation.

In contrast, comparative or analytic studies are designed for the investigation of causal relationships. The crucial aspect of these studies is the presence of a carefully selected control group matched for known relevant factors except those involved in the causal relationship under investigation. Because there's no deliberate intervention involved, they're collectively known as observational studies. Broadly speaking, they may be divided into cohort and case-control studies.

Cohort studies

The fundamental feature of cohort studies is that the groups under investigation are defined by their exposure to the causal factor.

In the simplest case, there are two groups, one comprising individuals exposed and the other those not exposed. For instance, if we're interested in determining whether or not oral contraceptives cause breast cancer, then we study two groups of women, one of which receives the pill, the other being the control group without exposure to the drug. The groups are subsequently observed over time to determine the occurrence in each group of the clinical outcome in question. In this case, subjects would be followed up for a suitable length of time during which all the cases of breast cancer in each group would be recorded.

Cohort studies may be retrospective or prospective. For example, a study performed today on a cohort of factory workers who were exposed to a chemical carcinogen in the 1960's in order to investigate the occurrence of bone cancer over the ensuing fifty years would be retrospective. On the other hand, if we recruited patients currently receiving a new drug and followed them for ten years to determine whether it increased the frequency of bone disease, this would be a prospective study.

Cohort Studies

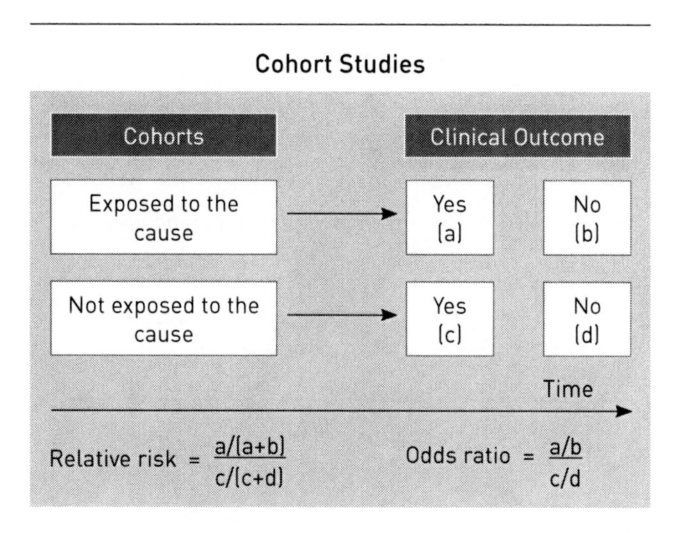

Cohort studies yield data that allow the estimation of the relative risk and odds ratio. Each of these is an expression involving a comparison of the outcome in the exposed group with that in the unexposed group. If there's no causal relationship between exposure and the outcome, then the relative risk or odds ratio will be close to unity. Values of greater than one – provided they are statistically significant – are interpreted as showing that the exposure promotes the outcome. Alternatively, values of less than one are said to indicate that the exposure protects against the outcome.

Case-control studies

Case-control studies are altogether different. They begin with patients with the disease and work backwards in an attempt to identify exposure to the suspected causal factor. Thus, they are, by definition, always retrospective.

The two study groups are defined in terms of the presence (cases) or absence (controls) of the disease and evidence is collected relating to exposure to the supposed cause in the past.

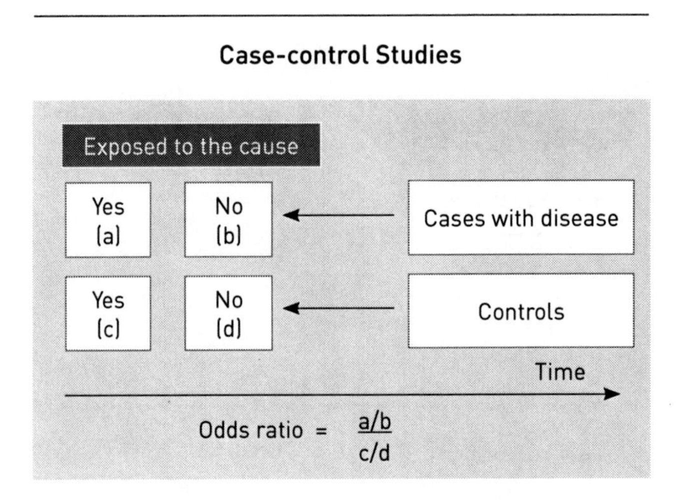

Case-control Studies

Case control studies are analysed using the odds ratio. The relative risk is inapplicable because of the direction of investigation from disease to exposure. Once again, a statistically significant odds ratio of greater than one is accepted as indicating the presence of a causal relationship.

The problem of bias

The objective of cohort and case-control studies is to compare the results for different groups and, if a statistically significant difference is detected, to infer a causal relationship between exposure and disease. In order to draw the correct inference, it's essential that the only difference between the two groups is that of exposure in cohort studies and the presence of disease in the case-control studies. However, it's generally accepted that all observational studies are subject to bias. There's always the possibility that other relevant factors for the outcome are not equally distributed between the groups.

The subject of bias in observational studies is confused and various classifications have been described.[2,3] Many of these are complex and, for the purposes of the present discussion, a simplified approach will be adopted.

Selection bias

The choice of controls is a crucial aspect of observational studies. For cohort studies, the aim is to select a group of individuals that match the exposed group as closely as possible for all variables apart from the exposure. For case-control studies, controls must match the cases as closely as possible for all variables apart from the presence of the disease. Selection bias results from a failure to match adequately the groups to be compared.

Data collection bias

Clearly, it's essential that the methods used to collect data regarding the end-point of the study are identical in each group. This applies to the assessment of disease in cohort studies and that of exposure in case-control studies. If possible, the researchers assessing the end-point should be blinded to the exposure in cohort studies and to the presence of the disease in case-control studies. Any difference in the assessment of the outcome between the groups in either type of study invalidates causal inference.

Data analysis bias

During the course of data analysis, bias may be introduced if the groups are treated differently. For example, a failure to handle losses to follow-up consistently in cohort studies results in differential losses between the groups producing bias.

Confounding

Confounding is present when both the supposed cause and the effect are associated with a third factor which is responsible – in whole or in part – for the difference in outcome detected between the groups. For example, when studying the relationship between oral contraceptives and vascular disease, smoking is a confounding variable because it is causally related to the development of vascular disease and is more prevalent in women who take the pill.

Provided the third factor is recognised – and this depends on the extent of background knowledge – measures may be taken, either at the stage of recruitment or in the analysis, to correct for possible confounding. Restriction involves excluding individuals with the known confounding variable from the study. Matching, on the other hand, includes individuals with the confounding factor but ensures that this is distributed equally between the two groups at the start of the study. This method, however, is limited in practice to just a few factors. Once the data have been collected, stratification or multivariate analysis may be used to adjust the observed difference for the effect of confounding factors. It's clear, though, that no methods are available for correcting for the presence of unknown confounding variables.

The Leap from Statistical Significance to Causation

The cardinal feature of cohort and case-control studies is that the finding of a statistically significant difference between the groups implies the presence of a causal relationship. The argument behind this is the belief that, if other differences have been excluded, then all that remains to explain the results is a causal relationship between exposure and disease. Of course, there can be no certainty that all other relevant differences have in fact been excluded and this weakness is inherent in all observational studies.

Nonetheless, it's become generally accepted that in certain contexts – for example, well-designed cohort or case-control studies with full attention to bias and confounding – a statistically significant difference establishes causation.

> "In epidemiology... we recognize the possible presence of a cause by its coincidence, beyond the bounds of chance, with the effect or change. That is to say, the suspect factor and the outcome are statistically associated." [4]

As already discussed, the statistical approach to research in epidemiology was a response to developments in the first half of the 20th century showing that cause and effect relationships in many spheres of medicine were far more complicated that hitherto supposed. Articles promoting the statistical approach to causation began to appear in the medical literature in the late 1950's.[5-8] But it was the publication in 1964 of the US Surgeon General's report on smoking and health – which included an account of the epidemiological criteria for the establishment of causation – that brought the matter to the fore.[9] Over the following decades, these criteria were revised by, amongst others, Bradford Hill,[10] Feinstein[11] and Susser.[4]

Criteria for causation in epidemiological studies

Strength of association

This refers to the closeness of the association between the cause and the effect, and is expressed in terms of the relative risk or odds ratio. In the 18th century, Percival Potts observed a strikingly high rate of cancer of the scrotum in chimney sweeps compared with that in other occupations. Given a relative risk of greater than 100, he reasonably inferred that exposure to the combustion products of coal caused the malignancy.[10] More than 200 years later, the strength of association remains the most important criterion in the epidemiological approach to causation. Bradford Hill, for example, had no doubts about its fundamental role. Referring to the marked increase in the risk of lung cancer in smokers, he commented:

> "...to explain the pronounced excess in cancer of the lung in any other environmental terms requires some feature of life so intimately linked with cigarette smoking and with the amount of cigarettes smoked that such a feature should be easily detectable. If we cannot detect it or reasonably infer a specific one, then in such circumstances I think we are reasonably entitled to reject the vague contention of the armchair critic 'you can't prove it, there may be such a feature'." [10]

It's well worth noting Bradford Hill's phrase "pronounced excess". His argument in support of the strength of association rests on the fact that the relative risks reported in the studies linking smoking to lung cancer were exceptionally high. As will be seen, this is of some importance but is, for the most part, ignored by modern day researchers obsessed with small relative risks.

Specificity

This criterion refers to the accuracy with which the occurrence of the cause predicts the occurrence of the effect and vice versa.[4] However, in most situations in medicine – where the cause is neither necessary nor sufficient for the effect – specificity is of only limited value in assisting with the identification of causal relationships.

Consistency

When an association between two variables is observed over a wide variety of different populations in different locations and at different times, the evidence in favour of a causal relationship is believed to be increased. The greater the variety of circumstances under which the association has been observed, the less likely it is that it's due to confounding.

The criterion of consistency is analogous to variative induction in science where experiments are conducted to test hypotheses under different conditions in order to exclude factors that might threaten any causal generalisation.[4,12]

Just as consistency is a strong criterion supporting causal inference, its absence argues against a cause and effect relationship.

Biological gradient

Epidemiological data that demonstrate an increase or decrease in the response variable proportional to changes in the predictor variable provide strong evidence of a causal relationship. Bradford Hill drew attention to the similarity between the biological gradient and the dose-response curves in physiology or pharmacology:

> "... the fact that the death rate from cancer of the lung rises linearly with the greater number of cigarettes smoked daily, adds a very great deal to the simpler evidence that cigarette smokers have a higher death rate than non-smokers... The clear dose-response

> curve admits of a simpler explanation and obviously puts the case in a clearer light." [10]

However, although the demonstration of a biological gradient is a powerful predictor of a cause and effect relationship, there may be difficulties with the interpretation of data due to non-linear relationships as well as threshold or saturation effects.

Coherence

This criterion refers to the degree to which a causal relationship may be accommodated within pre-existing knowledge and theory. The claims that prayer or touching the relics of a saint cures cancer would be dismissed out of hand because they are entirely at odds with everything that we know about medicine. If a study were to claim to prove either of these effects, the results would be dismissed on the grounds of a lack of coherence. There is, though, some debate about the interpretation of the term "coherence". It cannot, for example, be taken to mean complete consistency with what is already known about the subject for this would rule out any new finding and science would not progress. Coherence can't be interpreted too rigidly. There will always be a strong element of subjectivity with respect to this matter.

Epidemiological Criteria for Disease Causation

- Strength of association
- Specificity
- Consistency
- Biological gradient
- Coherence
- Experiments of nature
- Temporal priority

Experimental evidence

Sometimes, epidemiological data are the product of what are referred to as "natural experiments". The classical example is that of John Snow's observations of the cholera epidemics in London in the mid-19th century.[13] The 1849 epidemic occurred in areas of London supplied by the Southwark and Vauxhall Water Company and the Lambeth Water Company, both of which collected water from the Thames at sites polluted by sewage. Shortly afterwards, the Lambeth Water Company changed its source to a less polluted stretch of the river. In the subsequent 1854 epidemic, Snow observed that the rate of cholera in the area supplied by the Southwark and Vauxhall Water Company was more than eight times higher than that in the area supplied by the Lambeth Water Company. By changing its source of water away from the polluted regions of the Thames, the Lambeth Water Company unintentionally carried out an experiment and the data enabled Snow to confirm his hypothesis that cholera was transmitted by water polluted with sewage.

These "natural experiments" may provide strong evidence in favour of causal relationships. However, given that they are unintentional and uncontrolled, the data much be treated with caution.

Temporal priority

A cause must precede its effect. Eccentric physicists and science fiction writers may argue otherwise but, for the rest of us, we act and speak in line with the belief that a cause must occur before its effect, no matter how small the time interval involved. And the same holds true in medical research. It's certainly the case that establishing a temporal relationship may be difficult in chronic diseases studied retrospectively many years after exposure. But this is a practical matter, not a conceptual one. The basic point is this: once it has been shown that exposure occurred after the disease, the question of a causal relationship cannot be entertained. The most important role played by temporal priority is a negative one – to absolutely exclude a causal relationship when the disease is shown to occur before the exposure.

Applying the criteria for causation in epidemiology

In some situations, the epidemiological evidence in favour of a causal relationship is said to be strong. For example, the studies of smoking and lung cancer reported high relative risks, consistency of results over a broad range of different populations around the world and the presence of a definite biological gradient. While these data have been supported by animal studies and the demonstration of carcinogens in the combustion products of tobacco, they were believed to be sufficient on their own to establish that smoking causes lung cancer.

The finding of a lack of consistency and an absence of coherence with pre-existing knowledge and theory argue strongly against causation while the demonstration of a reversal of temporal priority militates against a causal relationship. However, the results of most epidemiological studies are far from being decisive one way or the other.

Bradford Hill emphasized that we can't prove causal relationships with epidemiological data.

> "What I do not believe – and this has been suggested – is that we can usefully lay down some hard-and-fast rules of evidence that must be obeyed before we can accept cause and effect. None of [the criteria] can bring indisputable evidence for or against the cause-and-effect hypothesis and none can be required as a sine qua non. What they can do, with greater or less strength, is to help us make up our minds on the fundamental question – is there any other way of explaining the set of facts before us, is there any other answer equally, or more, likely than cause and effect?" [10]

Thus, our judgment of the presence of a causal relationship should be grounded in the merits of the epidemiological data while acknowledging that whatever criteria are satisfied the judgment will be, at best, tentative and may be wrong.

But, for all the wise words and all the apparent emphasis on interpreting the set of criteria as a whole, the approach to epidemiological studies has focussed on a single item – that of the strength of association. Nowadays, this alone determines the presence of a causal relationship whilst the remainder of the criteria are relegated to mere mentions in the discussion section of published studies.

In many ways, the attention given to the strength of association is understandable. After all, relative risks and odds ratios are numerical values and may be subjected to statistical analysis. This isn't the case with many of the other criteria. However, whatever the reasons for giving prime importance to the criterion of strength, the consequences have been an unwelcome obsession with trivial differences manifested as small relative risks or odds ratios and a blind acceptance of causation when it is unwarranted.

When Percival Potts linked exposure to the combustion products of coal with cancer of the scrotum in 1775, he did so with evidence of a relative risk of approximately one hundred. When, in 1854, John Snow confirmed his hypothesis that exposure to polluted water was the source of cholera, he did so by observing a relative risk of eight in the context of an "experiment of nature". And when Doll and Hill identified the role of smoking in cancer of the lung in the 1950's, they did so with well-controlled observational studies showing a relative risk of between ten and thirty, as well as a definite biological gradient. Nobody now doubts these causal relationships.

All of this is a far cry from what happens nowadays. The research culture that puts so much stock in the statistical approach and the willingness to accept trivial relative risks and odds ratios has led to a proliferation of scare stories that pervade the news media, disseminate misinformation and bring medical research into disrepute.

Health Scare Stories

Modern societies are obsessed with health, obsessed with disease, in short, obsessed with all matters medical. This is reflected in the expansive coverage in newspapers and magazines, as well as on radio and television. The media interest drives our obsession and our obsession drives the media interest. Each feeds off the other. We want to read about, listen to, and watch anything to do with medicine. The media, in turn, have to satisfy the demand. It's fortunate, indeed, for the journalists and programme makers that there are such things as epidemiological studies. When the tales of medical mishaps run out, there's always a cohort study waiting to fill the void. And when there's a lull in the revelations of celebrities' addictions, eating disorders and cosmetic surgery, there'll be a case-control study ready for general release.

The proliferation of epidemiological studies is, in part, because they are relatively cheap, as well as being quick and easy to perform. In comparison with large randomised trials, they are much less expensive and aren't subject to the ethical restrictions that hinder interventional research. Case-control studies take relatively little time to complete – the investigators don't have to wait years after exposure for the disease to emerge. Furthermore, the availability of powerful computers to analyse the huge data-bases compiled over recent decades allows both cohort and case-control studies to be performed with minimal effort.

But it's not simply the almost unlimited stock of epidemiological studies that makes them so appealing to the media. It's also the fact that the conclusions of this type of research apply to large sections of the population. If eating beef-burgers causes heart attacks, then this seems to apply to everyone who visits a fast-food outlet. Journalists and broadcasters know this only too well. What they don't know – or rather, what they don't seem to know – is that these studies are utterly unreliable.

According to epidemiological research, if a man has fathered less than two children or works rotating shift patterns, then he's at increased risk of developing cancer of the prostate.[14,15] Eating bacon apparently increases the chance of bladder cancer[16] but so, for that matter, does drinking tap water.[17] Not only do mobile phones increase the risk of brain tumours[18] but, by some bizarre mechanism, they also reduce male fertility.[19] Anti-perspirants and deodorants are related to the development of breast cancer[20] while hair dyes cause lymphoma and lymphocytic leukaemia.[21-23] And eating beef-burgers more than once a week, we're told, is linked to asthma.[24] Even teaching your child to swim may not be such a good idea – it seems that exposure to chlorine may make them prone to hay fever.[25]

All of these reports were published in reputable journals; all of the claims are based on cohort or case-control studies; and all of the results were statistically significant. But does it really follow that men should throw their mobile phones away or that women should think twice about buying deodorants? Of course not. The evidence for doing so is flimsy if, indeed, it exists at all. To understand why this is the case, it's worth examining some of the more controversial claims made by epidemiologists recently.

Coffee and cancer of the pancreas

Consider, for instance, the saga of the link between coffee and pancreatic cancer. It began with a case-control study published in 1981 which reported an increased odds ratio of 1.8 (95% confidence interval 1.0-3.0).[26] Despite the unimpressive strength of association and borderline statistical significance, the study sparked concerns that coffee consumption might increase the risk of pancreatic cancer. Other case-control studies followed, some[27,28] reporting odds ratios of 2.3-2.5 while others[29-31] failing to show any significant effect. Furthermore, a large cohort study from Norway detected no association between coffee and pancreatic cancer.[32]

This example is instructive. It shows just how much influence epidemiological studies have – even when they produce results with trivial increases in odds ratios, they are taken seriously. But it also shows the weakness of this form of research. Paltry odds ratios may be enough to stimulate further research but the final product is a tangle of conflicting results. In the end, we're none the wiser; all that remains is rumour and myth that will find their way into textbooks of medicine for generations to come.

Red meat and malignant disease

Colorectal cancer

If we're to believe the experts, we should avoid eating meat if we wish to reduce our chances of developing cancer of the large bowel. But the data are far from convincing. On the one hand, a number of case-control[33-36] and cohort studies[37] have failed to identify any link between meat consumption and colorectal cancer. On the other, more recent cohort studies have suggested an association.[38-40] However, even amongst these positive reports, there's a lack of consistency. For example, in America, the consumption of meat increased the risk of both colonic and rectal cancer;[40] in Australia, it increased the risk only of rectal cancer;[38] whereas in Sweden, it had no effect on rectal cancer.[39]

As usual, when the data are inconsistent, the size of the risk is small. A recent meta-analysis reported an overall relative risk of colorectal cancer of 1.28 for red meat, with similar effects for processed meat.[41] But do these data really support a causal relationship between eating meat and cancer of the large bowel?

Breast cancer

Perhaps women should have further cause for concern about eating meat. A recent large cohort study from the United Kingdom reported that meat consumption was associated with an increased risk of breast cancer.[42] The results applied only to post-menopausal females with the highest risks observed in relation to processed meat (relative risk

1.64). Different results emerged from the USA where a larger cohort study reported that red meat increased the risk of breast cancer in pre-menopausal women but only for hormone receptor-positive tumours.[43] Interestingly, although the relative risk varied between 1.14 and 1.97 when the amount of meat consumed was taken into consideration, there was no clear dose-response. Earlier cohort and case-control studies produced conflicting results[44-47] while a pooled analysis of cohort studies involving more than 350,000 women showed no association between total meat consumption or red meat consumption and the risk of breast cancer.[48]

Once again, small increases in the relative risk and conflicting data hardly support the conclusion that eating meat is linked to breast cancer. But this didn't prevent the scare stories.

Passive smoking and lung cancer

Nowadays, it's widely accepted that passive smoking causes lung cancer. The campaign to ban smoking in public places was based on the belief that exposure to environmental tobacco smoke is responsible for at least some of the cases of lung cancer that occur in non-smokers. However, while there's a large body of evidence on the subject, its interpretation isn't straightforward and is further complicated by the polarised arguments of the anti-smoking movement and the tobacco industry.

Over the past 25 years, there have been more than 50 studies investigating the link between passive smoking and lung cancer. Taken individually, the data are inconsistent. Some studies report statistically significant associations[49] while others fail to show positive results.[50]

The relationship between the source of environmental tobacco smoke and the development of lung cancer is also inconsistent. Some studies report that exposure to passive smoking at home and at work are associated with lung cancer; others have found an association for only one of the two sources of exposure; yet others report negative findings in both settings. For example, in a recent study from China involving more than 65,000 women who had never smoked, exposure to environmental tobacco smoke in the home wasn't associated with an increased risk of lung cancer whereas there was a link between exposure at work and the disease although the statistical significance was borderline.[51]

While those with links to the tobacco industry emphasize the inconsistencies of the individual studies, those belonging to the anti-smoking movement stress the importance of looking at the entire body of evidence. A number of meta-analyses have been published and have tended to produce similar results with odds ratios in the region of 1.25.[52-55] This agreement, of course, isn't surprising given that they share many studies in common. However, the meta-analyses have been criticised on the grounds of possible publication bias leading to inflated estimates of risk.[56-57] Furthermore, Bayesian analysis of the same data sets indicates that conventional meta-analyses may have exaggerated the risks.[58] Despite these concerns, however, the general consensus amongst researchers is that exposure to environmental tobacco smoke, whether in the home or at work, increases the risk of lung cancer in non-smokers by approximately 25%.

There are, though, problems with accepting this pooled estimate of the risk of exposure to environmental tobacco smoke. Firstly, it must be remembered that it's based on epidemiological studies and, as such, is always open to the challenge that any statistically significant difference between the groups may be explained by reference to factors other than passive smoking. Secondly, the magnitude of the risk is extremely small.

Lung cancer in non-smokers is very uncommon.[50] Less than 5% of cases of lung cancer occur in non-smokers,[59,60] while studies in Europe and the USA suggest that the incidence of lung cancer in non-smokers is about 5-10/100,000 per year[55,61,62] with higher rates in females than in males. Given that the meta-analyses indicate an increase in risk of about 25%, passive smoking would be responsible for perhaps 1-2 cases of lung cancer per 100,000 of the population per year.

Accurately detecting such small effects is fraught with difficulty. This problem was highlighted in a report by the House of Lords Select Committee on Economic Affairs in 2006.[63] Sir Richard Peto, an eminent epidemiologist and expert in smoking-related diseases, was questioned about the data relating to passive smoking. His replies are very revealing.

> "... these risks are small and difficult to measure directly... measuring that risk reliably and directly is difficult... there is always going to be quite a lot of uncertainty about the magnitude of that risk... there is bound to be wide uncertainty when you are trying to measure risks like this... the trouble is that because these risks are small they are difficult to measure, for obvious reasons... it is difficult to measure small risks reliably... whatever those risks are, it is going to be difficult to measure them..." [63]

He agreed that he had been unwilling to quantify the risk from passive smoking. Instead, he reverted to his constant refrain that tobacco smoke is the most important cause of cancer in the world. But there was another telling aspect to his evidence. Time and again throughout the questioning, he fell back upon phrases such as,

> "... passive smoking must cause some risk of death [from cancer]... passive exposure to cigarette smoke must be producing some risk... I think there has got to be some risk... it has to be causing some risk... environmental tobacco smoke has to be causing some risk..." [63]

These, of course, are expressions to be used before any research has been carried out and are not appropriate after studies have been completed and published. They reflect belief, not scientific fact; opinion, not evidence.

From the testimony of Richard Peto, it's hard not to conclude that the link between passive smoking and lung cancer is simply unproven.

Despite a quarter of a century of research including numerous epidemiological studies, the data are insufficient for any definitive statement to be made. Yet somehow, the research community, the medical profession, the lay media, medical journals, politicians and their advisors, and civil servants in the Department of Health have been persuaded that exposure to environmental tobacco smoke causes lung cancer. Indeed, they were so convinced that the government was able to introduce legislation banning smoking in public places. It seems, though, that it was mistaken – or rather, that it had been misled. There was and is no firm evidence. This is certainly the conclusion drawn by the House of Lords Select Committee. The link between passive smoking and lung cancer is simply another scare story.

Epidemiology in Disrepute

Epidemiological studies are a good starting point for the investigation of statistics-based medical research. They may not be the "gold standard", but they are viewed by many as a source of reliable data. This is reflected in their position in the hierarchy of evidence, the large number of cohort and case-control studies published annually and the way in which their results influence the practice of medicine.

Some of the weaknesses of epidemiological studies are, however, well recognised. Firstly, the selection of controls will always be the subject of controversy. It's not simply a question of successfully matching all known factors related to the outcome, even if this were possible. Reliable causal inference depends on all factors, both known and unknown, being distributed equally and there's no reason to believe that this condition is satisfied in epidemiological studies. Secondly, unlike the situation in the experimental sciences and RCTs, there's no deliberate intervention to defend against the charge that the difference in outcome may due to something other than the causal factor under investigation.

Epidemiological studies may yield valuable information about causal relationships, particularly when a large relative risk or odds ratio is found. In most cases, however, the claims are unwarranted. Many of the problems stem directly from ignoring the advice given by Bradford Hill.[10] The consequences for epidemiology have been disastrous.

Emphasis on strength of association

When they were first compiled, the epidemiological criteria for the establishment of causation were intended to be used collectively and with a strong element of judgment.[10] However, under the influence of the statistical approach, the criteria have been curtailed, leaving the strength of association as the sole arbiter of a causal relationship. This development seriously reduces the reliability of causal inference.

The focus on small effects

The trend over recent decades to attribute importance to small effects reduces the reliability of causal inference. Genuine advances are associated with large effects.

Standardised Death Rates from Lung Cancer
Men aged >35 years (per 1000/year)

Non-smokers	Smokers			
	All	Mild	Moderate	Heavy
0.07	0.90	0.47	0.86	1.66

- Increased risk of lung cancer in heavy smokers v non-smokers = x24
- Dose-response effect present

Doll & Hill *BMJ* 1956

The link between smoking and lung cancer, for example, was identified by the finding of a relative risk of between ten and thirty.[1] Furthermore, there was a striking dose-response effect or biological gradient.

In contrast, the relative risk of lung cancer in relation to environmental tobacco smoke was found to be only 1.25. In other words, the risk of lung cancer, which is very uncommon in non-smokers, is increased by about one-quarter. As has been discussed, the ability of epidemiological studies to detect accurately such small increases in risk is highly debatable.

There is, though, a further aspect of small effects which requires consideration. Even if the risk is capable of accurate measurement, it's by no means clear that such a finding is useful in causal inference. Once again, Bradford Hill puts the matter succinctly:

> "Yet there are innumerable situations in which they [tests of significance] are totally unnecessary – because the difference is grotesquely obvious, because it is negligible, or because, whether it be formally significant or not, it is too small to be of any practical importance. What is worse, the glitter of the t table diverts attention from the inadequacies of the fare." [10]

We may be beguiled by statistics that purport to show a causal relationship. But there's much more to causation. In particular, when the effects are small, there's simply no point is performing statistical tests. Everything that needs to be said has already been shown by the data.

The strength of the association is not something absolute. Simply because the relative risk or odds ratio deviates from unity does not entail that it has causal import – even if the deviation is statistically significant. It is the magnitude of the strength of association taken in conjunction with all of the other criteria that justify tentative causal inference. This is the message that has been lost on the current generation of researchers.

Tarnished Reputation

The emphasis on small effects has a further undesirable consequence. Studies that report statistically significant relative risks or odds ratios close to unity are more likely to be contradicted by future studies than those reporting much larger effects. This accounts for the frequent finding of inconsistent results. The above examples of scare stories related to health demonstrate this clearly.

Contradictory results lead to the chopping and changing of recommendations regarding health matters from day to day. On any given topic, this engenders confusion. But worse, the constant exposure to so-called experts having to revise their guidance within a matter of months is greeted with ridicule.

> "Confused? Who wouldn't be? Big, small, short, fat, thin, breast, bottle, vegetarian, carnivore, coffee, tea, active, slothful – there's good or bad news (frequently both) depending on which day of the week you happen to have opened the papers." [64]

People are right to be sceptical about medical research. Cohort and case-control studies, and those who promote them, deserve the scorn heaped upon them. A sensible approach to epidemiological studies would be to ignore the results altogether.

References

1. Doll R, Hill AB. Lung cancer and other causes of death in relation to smoking. BMJ 1956;ii;1071-81.
2. Sackett DL. Bias in analytic research. J Chronic Dis 1979;32;51-63.
3. Grimes DA, Schulz KF. Bias and causal associations in observational research. Lancet 2002;359;248-52.

4. Susser M. Rules of inference in epidemiology. Regulatory Toxicology and Pharmacology 1986;6;116-128.
5. Lilienfeld AM. Epidemiological methods and inferences in studies of non-infectious diseases. Public Health Reports 1957;72;51-60.
6. Heubner RJ. Criteria for etiologic association of prevalent viruses with prevalent diseases: the virologist's dilemma. Ann N Y Acad Sci 1957;67;430.
7. Sartwell PE. On the methodology of investigation of etiologic factors in chronic diseases. J Chronic Dis 1960;11;61-63.
8. Yerushalmy J, Palmer CE. On the methodology of investigations of etiologic factors in chronic diseases. J Chronic Dis 1959;10;27.
9. Surgeon General's Advisory Committee on Smoking and Health: Smoking and Health 1964. United States Department of Health, Education and Welfare, Public Health Service Publication No. 1103. Chapter 3, Page 20.
10. Hill AB. The environment and disease: association or causation? Proc Roy Soc Med 1965;58;295-300.
11. Feinstein AR. Clinical biostatistics. Scientific standards vs. statistical association and biologic logic in the analysis of causation. Clin Pharmacol Ther 1979;25;481-492.
12. Penston J. Fiction and fantasy in medical research: the large-scale randomised trial. The London Press. London, 2003.
13. Snow J. Mode of Communication of Cholera. London, 2nd Ed. 1855. (Reprinted, New York, 1936)
14. Giwercman A, Richiardi A, Kaijser M, Ekbom A, Akre O. Reduced risk of prostate cancer in men who are childless as compared to those who have fathered a child: a population based case-control study. Int J Cancer 2005;115;994-7.
15. Kubo T, Ozasa K, Mikami K, Wakai K, Fujino Y, et al. Prospective cohort study of the risk of prostate cancer among rotating-shift workers: findings from the Japan collaborative cohort study. Am J Epidemiol 2006;164;549-55.
16. Michaud DS, Holick CN, Giovannucci E, Stampfer MJ. Meat intake and bladder cancer risk in 2 prospective cohort studies. Am J Clin Nutr 2006;84;1177-83.

17. Villaneuva CM, Cantor KP, King WD, Jaakkola JJ, Cordier S, et al. Total and specific fluid consumption as determinants of bladder cancer risk. Int J Cancer 2006;118;2040-7.
18. Hardell L, Carlberg M, Hansson MK. Pooled analysis of two case-control studies on the use of cellular and cordless telephones and the risk of benign brain tumours diagnosed during 1997-2003. Int J Oncol 2006;28;509-18.
19. Agarwal A, Deepinder F, Sharma RK, Ranga G, Li J. Effect of cell phone usage on semen analysis in men attending infertility clinic: an observational study. Fertil Steril 2008;89;124-8.
20. McGrath KG. An earlier age of breast cancer diagnosis related to more frequent use of antiperspirants/deodorants and underarm shaving. Eur J Cancer Prev 2003;12;479-85.
21. Milig L, Costantini AS, Benvenuti A, Veraldi A, Tumino R, et al. Personal use of hair dyes and hematolymphopoietic malignancies. Arch Environ Occup Health 2005;60;249-56.
22. Zhang Y, Holford TR, Leaderer B, Boyle P, Zahm SH, et al. Hair-coloring product use and risk of non-Hodgkin's lymphoma: a population-based case-control study in Connecticut. Am J Epidemiol 2004;159;148-54.
23. De Sanjose S, Benavente Y, Nieters A, Foretova L, Maynadie M, et al. Association between personal use of hair dyes and lymphoid neoplasms in Europe. Am J Epidemiol 2006;164;47-55.
24. Wickens K, Barry D, Friezema A, Rhodius R, Bone N, et al. Fast foods – are they a risk factor for asthma? Allergy 2005;60;1537-41.
25. Kohlhammer Y, Doring A, Schafer T, Wichmann HE, Heinrich J. Swimming pool attendance and hay fever rates in later life. Allergy 2006;61;1305-9.
26. MacMahon B, Yen S, Trichopoulos D, Warren K, Nardi G. Coffee and cancer of the pancreas. N Eng J Med 1981;304;630-3.
27. Lyon JL, Mahoney AW, French TK, Moser R. Coffee consumption and the risk of cancer of the exocrine pancreas: a case-control study in a low-risk population. Epidemiology 1992;3;164-70.
28. Gullo L, Pezzilli R, Morselli-Labate AM. Coffee and cancer of the pancreas: an Italian multicentre study. The Italian pancreatic Cancer Study Group. Pancreas 1995;11;223-9.

29. Wynder EL, Hall NE, Polansky M. Epidemiology of coffee and pancreatic cancer. Cancer Res 1983;43;3900-6.
30. Jain M, Howe GR, St Louis P, Miller AB. Coffee and alcohol as determinants of risk of pancreas cancer: a case-control study from Toronto. Int J Cancer 1991;47;384-9.
31. La Vecchia C, Liati P, Decarli A, Negri E, Franceschi S. Coffee consumption and risk of pancreatic cancer. Int J Cancer 1987;40;309-13.
32. Stensvold I, Jacobsen BK. Coffee and cancer: a prospective study of 43,000 Norwegian men and women. Cancer Causes Control 1994;5;401-8.
33. Steinmetz KA, Potter JD. Food-group consumption and colon cancer in the Adelaide Case-Control Study. II. Meat, poultry, seafood, dairy foods and eggs. Int J Cancer 1993;53;720-7.
34. Thun MJ, Calle EE, Namboodiri MM, Flanders WD, Coates RJ, et al. Risk factors for fatal colon cancer in a large prospective study. J Natl Cancer Inst 1992;84;1491-500.
35. Muscat JE, Wynder EL. The consumption of well-done red meat and the risk of colorectal cancer. Am J Public Health 1994;84;856-8.
36. Kampman E, Slattery ML, Bigler J, Leppert M, Samowitz W, et al. Meat consumption, genetic susceptibility, and colon cancer risk: a United States multicenter case-control study. Cancer Epidemiol Biomarkers Prev 1999;8;15-24.
37. Hsing AW, McLaughlin JK, Chow WH, Schuman LM, et al. Risk factors for colorectal cancer in a prospective study among US white men. Int J Cancer 1998;77;549-53.
38. English DR, McInnis RJ, Hodge AM, Hopper JL, Haydon AM, Giles GG. Red meat, chicken and fish consumption and risk of colorectal cancer. Cancer Epidemiol Biomarkers Prev 2004;13;1509-14.
39. Larsson SC, Rafter J, Holmberg L, Bergkvist L, Wolk A. Red meat consumption and risk of cancers of the proximal colon, distal colon and rectum: the Swedish Mammography Cohort. Int J Cancer 2005;113; 829-34.
40. Chao A, Thun MJ, Connell CJ, McCullough ML, Jacobs EJ, et al. Meat consumption and risk of colorectal cancer. JAMA 2005;293;172-82.

41. Larsson SC, Wolk A. Meat consumption and risk of colorectal cancer: a meta-analysis of prospective studies. Int J Cancer 2006;119;2657-64.
42. Taylor EF, Burley VJ, Greenwood DC, Cade JE. Meat consumption and risk of breast cancer in the UK Women's Cohort Study. Br J Cancer 2007;96;1139-46.
43. Cho E, Chen WY, Hunter DJ, Stampfer MJ, Colditz GA, et al. Red meat intake and risk of breast cancer among premenopausal women. Arch Intern Med 2006;166;2253-9.
44. Shannon J, Cook LS, Stanford JL. Dietary intake and risk of postmenopausal breast cancer (United States). Cancer Causes Control 2003;14;19-27.
45. Hermann S, Linseisen J, Chang-Claude J. Nutrition and breast cancer risk by age 50: a population-based case-control study in Germany. Nutr Cancer 2002;44;23-34.
46. Ambrosone CB, Freudenheim JL, Sinha R, Graham S, Marshall JR, et al. Breast cancer risk, meat consumption and N-acetyltransferase (NAT2) genetic polymorphisms. Int J Cancer 1998;75;825-30.
47. Holmes MD, Colditz GA, Hunter DJ, Hankinson SE, Rosner B, et al. Meat, fish and egg and risk of breast cancer. Int J Cancer 2003;104;221-7.
48. Missmer SA, Smith-Warner SA, Spiegelman D, Yaun SS,Adami HO, et al. Meat and dairy food consumption and breast cancer: a pooled analysis of cohort studies. Int J Epidemiol 2002;31;78-85.
49. Gorlova OY, Zhang Y, Schabath MB et al. Never smokers and lung cancer risk: a case-control study of epidemiological factors. Int J Cancer 2006;118;1798-804.
50. Vineis P, Airoldi L, Veglia P, et al. Environmental tobacco smoke and risk of respiratory cancer and chronic obstructive pulmonary disease in former smokers and never smokers in the EPIC prospective study. BMJ 2005;330;265-6.
51. Wen W, Shu XO, Gao Y-T, Yang G, Li Q, et al. Environmental tobacco smoke and mortality in Chinese women who have never smoked: prospective cohort study. BMJ 2006;333;376.
52. Hackshaw AK, Law MR, Wald NJ. The accumulated evidence on lung cancer and environmental tobacco smoke. BMJ 1997;315;980-8.

53. Taylor R, Cumming R, Woodward A, Black M. Passive smoking and lung cancer: a cumulative meta-analysis. Aust N Z J Public Health 2001;25; 203-11.
54. Stayner L, Bena J, Sasco AJ, Smith R, Steenland K, et al. Lung cancer risk and workplace exposure to environmental tobacco smoke. Am J Public Health 2007;97;545-51.
55. Boffetta P. Involuntary smoking and lung cancer. Scand J Work Environ Health 2002;28(S2);30-40.
56. Takagi H, Sekino S, Kato T, Matsuno Y, Umemoto T. Revisiting evidence on lung cancer and passive smoking: adjustment for publication bias by means of "trim and fill" algorithm. Lung Cancer 2006;51;245-6.
57. Copas JB, Shi JQ. Reanalysis of epidemiological evidence on lung cancer and passive smoking. BMJ 2000;320;417-8.
58. Tweedie RL, Scott DJ, Biggerstaff BJ, Mengersen KL. Bayesian meta-analysis, with application to studies of ETS and lung cancer. Lung Cancer 1996;14(Suppl 1);S171-94.
59. Capewell S, Sankaran R, Lamb D, McIntyre M, Sudlow MF. Lung cancer in lifelong non-smokers. Edinburgh Lung Cancer Group. Thorax 1991;46; 565-8.
60. Kabat GC, Wynder EL. Lung cancer in nonsmokers. Cancer 1984;53;1214-21.
61. Alipour S, Deschamps F, Lesage FX, Lebargy F. Estimation of annual incidence of lung cancer associated with work place exposure to passive smoking in France. J Occup Health 2006;48;329-31.
62. Wakelee HA, Chang ET, Gomez SL, Keegan TH, Feskanich D, et al. Lung cancer incidence in never smokers. J Clin Oncol 2007;25;472-8.
63. Select Committee on Economic Affairs, House of Lords. 2005-2006 session; Fifth Report. Chapter 5: Risk Management – Two cases. HL-183 II; pages 143-151.
64. Cochrane S. Guardian 1st March 2005.

IV

Casting Lots and Counting Funerals

To strike decisively against the statistical approach to medical research, we must target its flagship – the randomised controlled trial. But this isn't so easy. Randomised trials have two major advantages over observational studies, namely, deliberate intervention and random allocation of treatment. These characteristics, amongst others, are believed to protect against most of the challenges levelled against epidemiological studies.

The Evolution of the Randomised Controlled Trial

The importance of controls in clinical research has been recognised for centuries. If, as is often the case, the outcome is uncertain – for example, if some patients with the disease in question survive whilst others succumb – then controls are required to demonstrate the efficacy of treatment.

It's widely believed that the first controlled clinical trial was carried out by James Lind. In *A Treatise of the Scurvy* published in 1753, he presented his study in a strikingly similar format to that of modern day trials, beginning with a description of the patients.[1]

> "On the 20th of May 1747, I took twelve patients in the scurvy, on board the Salisbury at sea. Their cases were as similar as I could

> have them. They all in general had putrid gums, the spots and lassitude, with weakness of their knees. They lay together in one place, being a proper apartment for the sick in the fore-hold; and had one diet in common to all..." [1]

This was followed by a methods section in which he gave a detailed account of the intervention. Six treatments regimens were studied, each allocated to two patients.

> "Two of these were ordered each a quart of cider a day. Two others took twenty-five gutts of elixir vitriol three times a day... Two others took two spoonfuls of vinegar three times a day... Two of the worst patients... were put under a course of sea-water... Two others had each two oranges and one lemon given them every day... The two remaining patients, took the bigness of a nutmeg three times a day."[1]

Then, in a results section, he reported the clinical outcome in each group of patients.

> "The consequence was, that the most sudden and visible good effects were perceived from the use of the oranges and lemons; one of those who had taken them, being at the end of six days fit for duty... The other was the best recovered of any in his condition; and being now deemed pretty well, was appointed nurse to the rest of the sick." [1]

Finally, he presented his conclusions.

> "... the result of all my experiments was, that oranges and lemons were the most effectual remedies for this distemper at sea." [1]

But Lind had been fortunate. He had hit upon a treatment that worked – not one that marginally improved the symptoms, not one that benefited only some of the patients, but one that cured the disease in all who received it. Had this not been the case, he would have had little chance of showing such impressive results in just two patients. Moreover, he was familiar the natural history of the disease. Without this information, he couldn't have drawn the correct conclusions. Unless it was already known that the disease would persist without treatment, it could quite reasonably be argued that the sailors who recovered did so as a result of the natural history of the disease whilst those who remained sick had their recovery impaired by the noxious alternative therapies including sea water and vinegar. In other words, the inference that oranges and lemons cured scurvy depended crucially on information from historical controls.

It is somewhat of an irony that the advocates of evidence-based medicine – who acknowledge Lind's role in the development of clinical trials – shun research based on historical controls. And there's irony, too, in that Lind's study is a prime example in medical research where neither randomisation nor statistical analysis is required to establish efficacy of treatment. If there is no spontaneous resolution and the treatment works in all cases of the disease, randomised controlled trials are simply redundant.

The idea of controls, however, wasn't new. In 1752, the philosopher George Berkeley suggested how a therapeutic trial in patients with smallpox might be carried out.[2]

> "The experiment may be easily made, if an equal number of poor patients in the small-pox, were put into two hospitals at the same time of year, and provided with the same necessaries of diet and lodging, and, for further care, let the one have a tub of tar-water and an old woman, the other hospital, what attendance and drugs you please."[2]

The description of the intervention – a tub of tar and an old woman – is surely the most amusing and memorable in the annals of medical research. But, alongside it, there's much attention to detail in the formation of groups designed to be well matched in all respects apart from the treatment.

Lind's importance lies in the fact that he was the first to design, perform and publish a controlled clinical trial. His writings, though, reveal just how easy it is to introduce bias. While he recorded that the cases were as similar as possible, he also stated that two of the most serious cases were allocated to treatment with sea water. This raises the possibility that the choice of treatment may have been influenced by the severity of the disease. Here, in a nutshell, is the problem: how are we to select a control group that is as similar as possible to the patients receiving treatment? How can we be sure that there isn't some factor, other than the treatment, that's responsible for any difference in outcome between the groups?

The first hint of a solution to the problem appeared as long ago as 1662. In order to show that the medical practices of the time – in particular, blood letting and purgation – were responsible for more harm than good, van Helmont, a Flemish physician and chemist, proposed a controlled trial in which treatment was assigned to groups of patients on the basis of chance. [3]

> "Let us take out of the hospitals, out of the camps, or from elsewhere, 200 or 500 poor people, that have fevers, pleurisies, etc. Let us divide them in halfes, let us cast lots, that one halfe of them may fall to my share, and the other to yours; I will cure them without blood-letting and sensible evacuation; but do you do, as ye know... we shall see how many funerals both of us shall have: But let the reward of the contention or wager, be 300 Florens, deposited on both sides: here your business is decided." [3]

But the world of medical research in the 17th century wasn't ready for randomised controlled trials. His challenge to the authorities of the day was declined and an original idea was lost. It took more than two hundred years before medical research was to revisit the subject.

In 1898, Johannes Fibiger published the results of a therapeutic trial in Copenhagen which showed that the mortality from diphtheria was reduced by treating the patients with subcutaneous injections of serum.[4] It wasn't, however, the efficacy of treatment which made this study remarkable but rather Fibiger's awareness of the potential flaws in this kind of research and his solutions to these problems.[5] In particular, it was his method of selecting controls "*... to be as similar as possible to the ones treated with serum...*" [4] that was unique in the history of clinical trials. Although his words echo those of James Lind, his deeds were very different. Patients received either subcutaneous injections of serum plus standard care or standard care alone on the basis of alternate day allocation. Thus, the treatment each patient received depended only on the day they first attended the hospital – in a sense, it was determined by chance.

> "In many cases a trustworthy verdict can only be reached when a large number of randomly selected patients are treated with the new remedy and, at the same time, an equally large number of randomly selected patients are treated as usual." [4]

This should leave no one in any doubt as to Fibiger's place in the history of the development of clinical trials. His method of alternate day allocation may not be truly random, but his intention was clearly to randomise patients to different treatment groups. He surely deserves far more credit than he has received.[5]

Over the following fifty years or more, similar methods of alternate allocation of treatment were used in clinical trials.[6,7] There were also examples of allocation based of the toss of a coin[8] – harking back to van Helmont. But there was another development that was to be more influential than anything that had gone before. In the 1920s, RA Fisher described randomised experiments in agricultural research.[9] It didn't take long for medical researchers to see the relevance for therapeutic trials. Bradford Hill, for example, was one of the first, becoming a keen advocate of randomisation by the late 1930s.[10] The adoption of Fisher's methodology by medical researchers became inevitable. The first randomised trial, which investigated the efficacy of whooping cough immunisation, began in 1946 but didn't appear in print for a further five years.[11] Consequently, the MRC trial of streptomycin in pulmonary tuberculosis in 1948 became the first published randomised controlled trial in clinical research [12] – that is, of course, if we are to follow the convention of ignoring Johannes Fibiger.

The Objective of the Randomised Controlled Trial

The purpose of a RCT is to determine whether or not a particular treatment alters the outcome of patients. It is to identify a causal relationship between the treatment and the outcome. But, given the data, is causal inference justified? This is the fundamental question. There are, after all, other possible explanations for the observed difference.

Internal Validity

A clinical trial has internal validity if and only if

- inequalities between groups
- bias in assessment of outcome
- chance

have been excluded as possible explanations for the observed difference in outcome

Internal validity

Implicitly or explicitly, a checklist is used to ascertain whether causal inference is legitimate in any particular instance. If all three of the conditions are satisfied, then the study is said to have internal validity.

On the surface, it would appear that the first condition is addressed by randomisation, the second by blinding and the third by statistical analysis. But, as we will see, this rather simplistic approach hides considerable complexity. In respect of the various measures to achieve internal validity, there is considerable overlap in purpose and many interactions.

The conditions for internal validity that follow are designed to protect the integrity of causal inference reached on the basis of the data.

Condition 1: Excluding Inequalities between Groups

The aim of randomisation is the equal distribution of all factors relevant to the outcome between the groups at the start of the trial. But this equal distribution must be maintained throughout the study.

There are various points during the study where randomisation may be disrupted including, for example, the handling of losses to follow-up and the statistical analysis. Furthermore, knowledge of treatment allocation may lead to differences in the way the patients are managed, thus introducing new inequalities between the groups that may be relevant to the outcome.

Condition 1
Excluding inequalities between the groups

Purpose	Mechanisms
Formation of equal groups	• Randomisation • Allocation concealment
Preservation of equal groups	• Blinding • Intention-to-treat • Avoiding particular statistical analyses

In order to satisfy the first condition for internal validity, it's essential that the groups have an equal distribution of relevant factors throughout the study up to the point when inferences are drawn about the difference in outcome between the groups.

Formation of Equal Groups

The formation of equal groups at the start of the study depends on the generation of a random sequence and the avoidance of any bias in applying this sequence to the allocation of treatment to individual patients.

Randomisation

Allocating patients to one group or another entirely on the basis of chance is believed to lead to the formation of groups that are equal in terms of all of the variables related to the outcome – both known and unknown. This is thought to be achieved by randomisation. In the present context, "random" is a technical term referring to the characteristic that the treatment allocation for any individual participant cannot be predicted.[13,14] The generation of a genuinely random sequence is mandatory and this may be achieved using either random number tables or a computer-generated random sequence.

In addition to forming equal groups, randomisation also has an important role in ensuring that the conditions for statistical tests are satisfied. This is discussed in chapter VI.

Although, in theory, randomisation offers a solution to the problem of controls, there are many difficulties associated with its implementation in practice.

(a) Omission of details of randomisation

Accurate descriptions of how randomisation was achieved are frequently missing from published RCTs. In fact, there's a failure to specify the method of randomisation in the majority of clinical trials.[15-22] We certainly can't assume that the allocation of treatment was a truly random process – one report suggested that 5% of supposedly randomised trials actually used non-randomised methods.[20]

Problems with Randomisation

- Inadequate reporting
- Pseudo-randomisation
- Unequal numbers in groups
- Unequal distribution of relevant factors
- Deliberate manipulation of randomisation procedure

(b) Pseudo-randomisation

Some clinical trials use methods of treatment allocation that, while believed to be random, are in fact either predictable or capable of being manipulated so as to make them predictable.

Alternate allocation of treatment is clearly predictable. Knowledge of the next treatment gives the investigators the opportunity to delay recruitment of a particular patient until what they believe to be a more suitable treatment is scheduled. Although the toss of a coin is random, it is also open to manipulation.

Alternate allocation of treatment, tossing a coin, deciding on the groups according to date of birth and other similar methods fail to eliminate predictability and thus are not truly random. It's not surprising, therefore, that pseudo-randomisation has been associated with bias in clinical trials.[23-26]

(c) Formation of unequal groups

Randomisation may yield either unequal numbers of patients or an unequal distribution of factors relevant to the outcome simply as a result of chance. It's generally accepted that, in large studies with more than 200 participants, the differences are unlikely to be important. However, inequalities should be avoided in smaller studies and a variety of different methods are available.[13]

To achieve equal numbers of patients in each group, allocation of treatment may be divided into blocks. For example, if each block comprises treatment for eight patients, then four patients will be randomly allocated to the active drug and four to placebo. Blocking, however, impairs the unpredictability of random allocation. If the trial isn't blinded, or if the active drug produces common and easily recognised side-effects, the investigator will know what treatments have already been allocated within that block and, given that he knows the number in each block, he will be able to predict which treatments remain. Consequently, selection bias may occur.[13,27] Although this problem may be lessened by varying the size of the blocks, there's no guarantee that this will be successful.[28]

Inequality in the distribution of relevant factors is more important than that of the number of patients in each group. As Austin Bradford Hill made clear, the purpose of randomisation is "*...to ensure beforehand that, as far as possible, the control and the treated groups are the same in all relevant respects.*"[10] If it fails in this objective, it's of little value. RCTs usually provide a table showing the proportion of patients in each group with various characteristics – for example, age, sex, co-existent disease, pre-trial medication and smoking habits. Baseline imbalance – that is, differences between the groups – is commonly observed although it's generally dismissed as being of little importance. However, although the differences in baseline characteristics are usually small, they may be of a similar magnitude to the difference in outcome observed in large-scale RCTs. It's only to be expected, therefore, that the findings of multi-centre randomised trials – including, for instance, the HOPE study and the LIFE study – have been challenged on the grounds of baseline imbalance.[29-32] And, of course, it should be remembered that baseline data relate to only a small number of factors relevant to the outcome. Many others are simply unknown.

Baseline imbalance may be reduced by restricted randomisation using stratification in blocks. But it's complicated, limited to a small number of factors and may introduce bias. This is of concern, particularly as restricted randomisation is often unreported and may lead to unsuspected selection bias.[20,33]

(d) Evidence of manipulation of randomisation

Randomisation, when carried out correctly, shouldn't be expected to produce identical numbers of patients in each of the treatment groups. In fact, the opposite is the case. Yet, surprisingly, trials that are reported as being randomised yield groups with equal numbers of patients more often than would be expected by chance.[18,20,21] Studies have shown that between a half and three-quarters of trials using simple randomisation recorded equal numbers – results that are inconsistent with the outcome of a truly random process.[34] There are reports, too, of deliberate attempts to interfere with randomisation in order to manipulate the outcome of RCTs.[23,27,35]

These findings challenge the foundations of RCTs and bring into question their internal validity. However, as with fraud in medical research in general, the frequency is unknown.

Allocation concealment

It's clear that if an investigator knows the next treatment, he may choose to delay the recruitment of a particular patient until a different treatment is scheduled. Thus, even if the sequence generated is random, the groups may not be equal because the allocation of treatment has been manipulated. Allocation concealment is designed to prevent those recruiting patients from knowing the next treatment before an individual is enrolled in the study. Its aim is to avoid selection bias.[14,23]

Various methods have been used to conceal allocation including sequentially numbered sealed envelopes or containers, and central randomisation.[36] Ideally, those involved in either generating the randomised sequence or allocating the treatments should not participate in the recruitment of patients. Central randomisation by telephone is the preferred option nowadays with investigators providing details of the patient before being given the treatment allocation.[14,36]

As with randomisation, errors and omissions related to allocation concealment are not uncommon.

(a) Failure to report details of allocation concealment

Evidence from literature reviews suggests that adequate details about allocation concealment are omitted in up to three-quarters of published randomised trials.[18,20-22,37-40] While some reports indicate that missing information doesn't necessarily imply inadequate allocation concealment,[41] others suggest that the failure to report details is closely associated with poor allocation concealment in practice.[39] RCTs which fail to disclose sufficient details should be treated with caution.

(b) Effects of inadequate allocation concealment

By providing investigators with knowledge of the next treatment, failure of allocation concealment destroys randomisation and produces groups that differ from one another in more than just the treatment.[23,27] In terms of the internal validity of RCTs, allocation concealment is considered by some to be of more importance than either the reliable generation of a random sequence or successful blinding.[23,35]

Studies associated with inadequate allocation concealment tend to produce larger treatment effects than those with successful concealment, the difference in treatment effects being reported to be as high as 40%. While some studies don't support this conclusion,[42,43] the evidence suggests that failure of allocation concealment leads to selection bias associated with exaggerated treatment effects.[23-25,35,40,44,45]

Problems with Allocation Concealment

- Inadequate reporting
- Success threatened by block design or absence of blinding
- Deliberate manipulation

(c) Effect of block randomisation on allocation concealment

As we have seen, trial design involving randomisation in blocks allows prediction of allocation in patients towards the end of each block. This occurs when the investigators are aware of the earlier treatments, either because the trial is not blinded or because of the occurrence of well-recognised and common side effects. Successful blinding, however, helps to protect allocation concealment when block randomisation is used.

(d) Deliberate undermining of allocation concealment

Investigators may deliberately undermine randomisation and allocation concealment.[23-25,27,35,46] Although the frequency is unknown, many researchers are aware of instances of research misconduct in relation to allocation concealment.[27,36,47,48] Schulz and Grimes, for instance, document a litany of different offences in this context.[36]

Preservation of Equal Groups

Let's accept that randomisation and allocation concealment deliver equally matched groups. This is only the beginning of the story. The equal distribution of factors relevant to the outcome must be protected throughout the study. But this may be disrupted by a failure of blinding, the omission of some randomised patients from the analysis and faulty statistical techniques.

Problems with Preservation of Randomisation

- Absence or failure of blinding
- Inadequate handling of withdrawals and losses to follow-up
- Flawed statistical techniques

Blinding

The use of double-blind administration of treatment is important in the preservation of equal groups throughout the study. Knowledge of the treatment may influence the way in which investigators manage patients during the study. This may lead to differences between the groups in respect of additional medication, investigations, referral for surgery, and decisions about withdrawal from the study. The effect is to create new differences between the previously well-matched groups that affect the outcome.

Effects of losses from final analysis

Participants may be deliberately removed from a trial for a variety of reasons. They may have been inappropriately recruited to the study and found after randomisation to have failed to meet the selection criteria. There may have been violations of the study protocol, such as a failure to attend for scheduled investigations or the use of other prohibited medication. They may have developed unrelated serious disease during the study or they may have become pregnant. And, of course, adverse drug reactions often result in patients leaving the study prematurely. In all of these cases, the decision to withdraw patients from a trial is made by the investigators. However, patients may also be lost from follow-up due to their own actions. For example, they may choose not to participate in the trial any longer or they may move away to a different location making follow-up impossible.

Losses must be kept to a minimum because failure to include all patients in the final analysis leads to bias. Intention-to-treat analysis includes all individuals randomised to trial medication even if they violate the protocol or are withdrawn from the study for other reasons. However, it's often the case that the total number of patients in the final analysis falls short of the number randomised at the start of the study. In this situation, it's important that investigators accurately report the number of missing patients and provide sufficient details to assist with interpretation. Such data, though, are frequently omitted.[38,49-51] Interestingly, even when RCTs claim to include all patients in an intention-to-treat analysis, further scrutiny shows that this is often not the case [51] and that these studies have other methodological flaws.[52]

Intention-to-treat analysis avoids the disruption of randomisation associated with the exclusion of patients.[53,54] While there's debate about the matter – with some reports playing down the importance [23,55] – the general view is that incomplete analysis of all randomised patients leads to bias.[56-60]

In principle, we can never be certain that the reasons for withdrawal or loss to follow-up are unrelated to the outcome of the study. In practice, it's often clear that the two are related. Patients may be withdrawn from a study because of poor symptom response or the development of adverse drug reactions; they may be lost to follow-up because they died from the disease. It's easy to see how a failure to include all randomised patients in the final analysis leads to an overestimation of treatment effects.[59,60] If internal validity is to be achieved, losses must be minimised and handled correctly.

Disruption due to statistical analysis

The treatment effect in subgroups of the study population is commonly part of the data analysis of randomised controlled trials. For example, in studies of the effect of drugs in the prevention of cardiovascular disease, not only is the overall outcome reported but also that for males and females, smokers and non-smokers, diabetics and non-diabetics, etc. The problem is, of course, that separating the groups receiving active drug or placebo each into males and females or smokers and non-smokers breaks the randomisation sequence. Subgroups are selected on the basis of certain characteristics and not by randomisation.

Thus, subgroup analysis disrupts the equal distribution of variables established by randomisation.[61,62] Any inference regarding the treatment effect in subgroups is, therefore, subject to challenge. This is discussed in more detail in Condition 3.

Condition 2: Excluding Bias in Assessment of Outcome

The trial outcome

Nowadays, RCTs, especially those involving large numbers of patients, usually study more than one outcome or end-point. The primary end-point is selected by the investigators to measure what they consider to be the most important outcome. It's also used in the calculation of the number of patients needed to be recruited to the study in order to obtain statistical significance. End-points, whether primary or secondary, may be simple, complex or composite. A simple end-point measures a single outcome whereas composite end-points include multiple outcomes and are discussed in more detail in Chapter V.

In the present context, it's of more relevance to classify the outcome into hard and soft end-points. The hardest of all end-points is usually accepted to be all-cause mortality.[45] Often, "cause-specific" mortality is preferred but, as the cause of death may be disputed, this is a somewhat less reliable end-point. At first glance, it may seem that myocardial infarction, for example, is a hard end-point but this isn't always the case. Most physicians would accept that this has occurred when a patient has classical ischaemic chest pain accompanied by ST-segment elevation with a typical distribution on the ECG and a raised troponin level. But what of a patient who has an atypical clinical presentation and elevated enzymes together with equivocal ECG changes? As in much of medicine, grey areas are common and judgment is required on the part of clinicians and investigators.

Soft end-points are usually subjective, involving alterations in symptoms but without observable changes either on examination or with respect to the results of clinical tests. Examples include the relief of pain in irritable bowel syndrome, the improvement in well-being in chronic fatigue syndrome or the lessening of depression in psychiatric illness. Such changes, even with the assistance of validated scales of symptoms, depend entirely on the account given by each individual patient.

It's clear, then, that there's a spectrum of outcomes assessed in clinical trials which range from hard "objective" end-points to soft "subjective" end-points. The terms, however, are relative and there's no rigid demarcation between them. Nonetheless, they're useful when considering the question of bias in the assessment of the outcomes of clinical trials.

Blinding

Blinding is the primary means by which bias in the assessment of the outcome is avoided. The idea of keeping subjects and investigators unaware of the intervention has a long history in various fields of science.

Purposes of Blinding

- Prevention of bias in the assessment of the outcome
- Protection against disruption of allocation concealment in trials using block randomisation
- Maintenance of equal distribution of variables throughout the trial
- Prevention of bias during data analysis

The topic of blinding is often confused by the terminology. An *open*, or *non-blinded*, study is one in which participants and investigators know the treatment received. A *single-blind* study involves either patients or investigators – usually the former – being unaware of the treatment. The term *double-blind*, although commonly used, may create confusion if not clearly defined. It usually indicates that neither patients nor investigators know the treatment received. However, blinding may also refer to those who assess the outcome or those who analyse the data. Thus, terms such as "triple-blind" and even "quadruple-blind" have appeared in the literature.[63]

Blinding has a number of important functions in randomised controlled trials and some of these have been discussed already. Traditionally, the purpose of blinding is to prevent any of those involved in the trial from introducing bias into the assessment of the outcome. Both patients and investigators may be influenced by the knowledge of treatment allocation. In general, it's believed that blinding is particularly valuable in trials with soft end-points although the so-called harder end-points are not immune to bias. Although the emphasis is usually placed upon the assessment of the outcome, bias may also occur during data analysis. For example, decisions regarding the handling of withdrawals and drop-outs may be influenced by knowledge of the treatment received.

Limitations to blinding

In many clinical situations, double-blind allocation of treatment isn't possible. This is the case, for example, with surgical operations, physiotherapy, exercise regimens and behavioural therapy. When it comes to most therapeutic trials, though, the circumstances would appear to be entirely suited to the double-blind technique. But this is deceptive.

There are numerous ways in which blinding may fail.[14,64] To begin with, any detectable differences between the active drug and placebo may disclose treatment allocation to either the patients or the investigators.[65,66] Efforts must be made to ensure that the tablets or capsules in the active treatment group are identical in respect of appearance (size, shape and colour), taste and smell to those of the placebo group.

But even if it were possible to produce identical preparations, other problems may thwart the attempt to blind patients and investigators to treatment. Certain drugs produce changes in the colour of urine; rifampicin, for example, causes an orange discolouration. Others – for instance, iron and bismuth compounds – colour the stools black. Physiological changes may also disclose treatment; beta-blockers cause bradycardia that's easily detected on examination. Then, of course, there are side-effects which readily inform of the presence of the active drug; tremor with salbutamol, dry mouth with anticholinergics, photosensitivity with chloroquine and postural hypotension with anti-hypertensive agents. Finally, the response to treatment itself – in particular, the alleviation of chronic symptoms early in the course of the trial – may offer evidence that the active drug has been prescribed.[67]

Problems with Blinding

- Limitations
  - Clinical situation
  - Preparation of placebo to match drug
  - Physiological effects
  - Side effects
- Inadequate reporting
- Deliberate interference with blinding

Inadequate reporting

The reporting of blinding is frequently unsatisfactory with studies indicating that it's inadequate in up to half of clinical trials.[21,37,68,69] Given the confusions surrounding the terminology and the availability of different techniques, a detailed description of the methods used to disguise the treatment is required. Yet, it's often the case that studies merely report that double-blind allocation was used or, worse, omit any mention of blinding altogether.[21,37,52,70]

The importance of blinding

There is considerable disagreement regarding the requirement for blinding in clinical trials. Some studies suggest that there's no difference in treatment effects between trials with and those without blinding – in other words, that blinding doesn't affect the outcome.[42,43] Not only is this counterintuitive, but it's not supported by other studies which indicate that blinding reduces bias in RCTs.[23,35,44,71-74] A recent study which analysed data from 1,346 trials reported that estimates of treatment effects were exaggerated when subjective end-points were assessed without binding but this finding wasn't present when hard end-points were involved.[45]

Many of the arguments against the need for blinding focus on the view that it's not required for hard end-points. While this assumes that such outcomes aren't open to misinterpretation or manipulation – which isn't the case – it also neglects that fact that blinding plays other important roles in satisfying the conditions for internal validity.

Deliberate interference with blinding

As noted earlier, attempts to interfere with allocation concealment are well documented in the literature. When this occurs in double-blind trials, it obviously involves breaking the blinding. Not only does this wreck allocation concealment, but also it further disrupts the equal distribution of relevant factors during the study as well as leading to bias in the assessment of the outcome.

However, blinding may also be deliberately broken during the study after successful treatment allocation. Investigators have ready access to the tablets or capsules – for example, they handle medication both to assess compliance and provide treatment for the next period – and hence have ample opportunity to obtain samples of the medication in order to determine which treatment any given patient is receiving.

Condition 3: Excluding Chance

The purpose of statistical analysis is to determine whether the difference in outcome between the groups is to be attributed to chance. To many, this may seem to be the most straightforward part of RCTs. Statistical analysis is often taken to be an automatic process whereby the raw data are fed into a computer to yield a P-value or confidence interval. And, within mainstream medical statistics, there is, in general, a consensus about how data should be analysed. However, as will be discussed in chapter VI, there are important disputes in the wider community of statisticians about fundamental aspects of their subject. Here, though, we will focus on a particular example of statistical analysis that is the source of much disagreement and, especially when it is used incorrectly, leads to flawed statistical significance which adversely affects internal validity.

Subgroup analysis

A common problem in the statistical analysis of large RCTs relates to multiple comparisons.[62,75] These include comparisons of the effects of treatment on multiple end-points, of the effects of multiple treatments on a single end-point, and of the effects of treatment in different subgroups of patients.[75] It's generally acknowledged that statistically significant differences detected in multiple comparisons must be viewed with suspicion.[75-77]

Given that large-scale RCTs involve heterogeneous study populations, it's always open to doubt as to whether the overall result applies to particular kinds of patients. Thus, there's a temptation to analyse the treatment effects in different subgroups.[62] This type of analysis is considered valuable because it may show that the results are applicable to all patients studied or that the treatment is ineffective in particular subgroups, hence avoiding unnecessary medication. There are, though, less charitable explanations for the widespread use of subgroup analysis. When a pharmaceutical company embarks on a large clinical trial, it not only involves great expense but places their product at risk. Including subgroup analysis lessens this risk; while the overall result may not be favourable, positive results in particular groups of patients may come to the rescue – it's rather like an insurance policy. Thus, subgroup analysis turns out to be a useful marketing ploy.

Whatever the reasons behind the subgroup analysis, it's certainly rife. Not only is it used in most RCTs, but it often involves dozens of different comparisons.[76,78,79] It's not always clear, though, how many comparisons have actually been made. There's evidence of selective reporting, with comparisons yielding positive results included in the

Problems with Subgroup Analysis

- Inadequate or selective reporting
- Failure to use correct techniques (tests of interaction)
- False positives
- False negatives
- Disruption of randomisation
- Undesirable clinical consequences

publication while the remainder are omitted.[75,80-82] This practice hinders interpretation of the findings and leads to bias in future meta-analyses.[82] And there are many other problems.

False positives

Subgroup analysis, like all multiple comparisons, may lead to false positive findings. [61,76,83-86] This follows from basic probability theory. Each comparison is an attempt to detect a difference and the more attempts that are made, the greater the probability that a difference will be detected simply due to chance. In the ISIS-2 study,[87] for example, the overall results showed a reduction in mortality from myocardial infarction with aspirin yet subgroup analysis suggested that the drug was of no benefit to those born under the sign of Gemini or Libra.

When a study reports no overall effect, subgroup analysis is particularly vulnerable to producing the wrong conclusions.[75,84-86] This is especially true with data dredging when the comparisons are ad hoc rather than specified beforehand in the study protocol.[75,76] Here, the results of subgroup analysis should be rejected.

False positive findings stem from a faulty statistical analysis that looks for treatment effects separately in each subgroup.[76] The correct approach is to use a test of interaction which determines whether the treatment effect differs between the subgroups.[86] However, only a minority of studies using subgroup analysis report tests of interaction.[76]

False negatives

The statistical analysis of RCTs centres on the primary end-point. It's the expected size of the difference in this outcome in the total study population that, amongst other factors, determines the size of the study population. All things being equal, any reduction in the sample size lessens the power to identify differences as being statistically significant. It follows, therefore, that subgroups analysis – which, by definition, reduces the size of the groups included in the comparison – is less able to detect statistically significant differences. This is the source of false negatives.

Studies show that false negatives are common in subgroup analysis.[61,76,84-86] Thus, care is required in interpreting negative subgroup comparisons, particularly in the presence of an established overall effect.

Interference with randomisation

When subgroup analysis is performed, individuals are selected for each subgroup on the basis of the presence or absence of a particular characteristic – for example, age, gender, or smoking, etc. This disrupts randomisation.[61,62] As a consequence, it can't be assumed that the subgroups are equally matched in terms of the distribution of other factors relevant to the outcome. Inevitably, internal validity is flawed. In addition, given that statistical tests depend on independent randomised samples, the results of subgroup analysis are further brought into question.

Undesirable consequences of subgroup analysis

It may reasonably be argued that subgroup analysis should be abandoned. If it fails to show any effect, this can't be assumed to be the case as false negatives are only to be expected. Equally, positive results are open to doubt. Furthermore, even if the correct statistical tests have been carried out, the disruption of randomisation weakens any causal inference.

Rothwell, in a comprehensive account of the subject, presented an extensive list of examples which demonstrate the clinical problems resulting from incorrect conclusions drawn from subgroups analysis.[62] False positive findings may lead to the administration of unnecessary treatment with risks of adverse drug reactions while false negative results may prevent patients from receiving medication that would otherwise be of benefit to them.

Finally, there's an important lesson to be learnt from the current fashion for subgroup analysis: despite the involvement of statisticians, the statistical analysis of data from large RCTs may be flawed.

More fundamental problems with statistical analysis of RCTs

Subgroup analysis provides a good example of the way in which statistical methods may deliver unreliable conclusions and threaten internal validity. But there are more general problems related to statistical analysis in medical research.

Behind the façade of agreement, serious disputes about the fundamentals of statistics are to be found. This isn't at all unexpected. Statistics is based on probability and, given that there are various theories of probability,[88] it's inevitable that there will be variety of different approaches to statistics. For example, conventional statistics – as used in medical research, psychology and the social sciences – is based on the frequentist theory of probability while, in recent times, there has been increasing interest in Bayesian statistics. These two very different approaches often produce different statistical analyses of the same data sets leading to conflicting conclusions about the outcome of experiments or clinical trials. But how are we to decide which conclusions are to be accepted? These important matters are discussed in chapter VI.

Problems with Statistical Analysis

- Faulty statistical techniques (e.g. subgroup analysis)
- Uncertainties about statistical theory
- Questions about statistical causation

At an even deeper level, there's the question of the legitimacy of the statistical approach to causation. This is taken for granted. Yet the notion that a small difference in outcome between groups in a RCT justifies causal inference is far from being straightforward. This issue is addressed in chapters X and XI.

For the time being, it's sufficient to say that the reliance on statistics to exclude chance as an explanation for the finding of differences in outcome between the groups in RCTs is, at the very least, questionable.

Conclusions

Randomisation has a strong appeal. In theory, it offers a solution to the long recognised problem of selecting groups that are equally matched in the distribution of all factors related to the outcome. This is its primary role. It also satisfies a requirement for conventional statistical tests. These two functions, though, should be viewed separately. It's worth recalling that the first published randomised trial in 1948 contained no statistical tests.[12] It was only later that statistical analysis began to form part of RCTs. As the years passed and clinical trials focused on detecting ever smaller treatment effects, the requirement for statistical tests became essential.

Poor reporting of RCTs is endemic. This has been extensively documented [15-18,20,37,38,48,49] and, although there's some evidence of improvements in the quality of reporting, the problem persists.[49,89-91]

Inadequate or missing information about the various components doesn't necessarily entail that a RCT fails to satisfy the conditions for internal validity. However, not only does it preclude any reliable interpretation of the data but it's also associated with a failure to carry out correctly procedures that are essential for internal validity.[39]

The problems with published medical research have been recognised for many years. In 1986, Rennie wrote scathingly about the subject[92] and, despite efforts to improve the situation with respect to RCTs, criticisms continue.[93,94] As the methodology is refined with new checks and balances introduced to improve internal validity, all that seems to happen is that clinical trials become more complex, more opaque and more unwieldy. Every adjustment and every added component merely deliver new points of weakness creating yet more grounds for concern about the reliability of the results and the legitimacy of the conclusions.

Nonetheless, the RCT reigns supreme in the hierarchy of medical research. It's trusted by drug regulatory authorities, researchers and practicing physicians to deliver reliable evidence on which to base treatment. But, as has been shown, when it's closely examined, it fails to live up to expectations. This chapter has concentrated on what might be called the mechanics of the RCT – randomisation, allocation concealment, blinding, handling of withdrawals and statistical analysis – and each of these processes has been found wanting.

There's no guarantee that the conditions for internal validity have been satisfied. Although randomisation and allocation concealment may have been performed to the highest standards, the groups may not be equally matched. The trial may have been carried out in a double-blind fashion, but the treatments may have been disclosed, resulting in newly introduced inequalities between the groups and bias in the assessment of the outcome. The handling of withdrawals and drop-outs, regardless of reported intention-to-treat analysis, may have been inadequate. And the statistical analysis used may have been faulty. The evidence indicates that innocent mistakes, culpable ignorance and deliberate acts of research misconduct combine to raise serious questions about the internal validity of randomised controlled trials.

RCTs in Practice

	Inadequate reporting	Evidence of flaws
Randomisation	+	+
Allocation concealment	+	+
Blinding	+	+
Handling of withdrawals and losses to follow-up	+	+
Statistical analysis	+	+

Only the most trenchant advocates of statistics-based research would believe that it's unproblematic. On the contrary, any impartial observer would be forced to conclude that it's riddled with flaws and that, in any particular instance, we can have little confidence that the conclusions of a RCT are valid.

But this is not the end of the matter. As will be discussed in subsequent chapters, there are other serious problems that face anyone who considers using the conclusions of RCTs to guide them in the management of patients.

References

1. Lind J. *A Treatise of the Scurvy.* Printed by Sands, Murray and Cochran. Edinburgh, 1753.
2. Berkeley G. A second letter to Thomas Priori on the virtues of tar-water. In: *The Works of George Berkeley.* Dublin. John Exshaw, 1784. Vol I.

3. Van Helmont JB, *Oriatrike, or physick refined: the common errors therein refuted and the whole art reformed and rectified.* Lodowick-Loyd. London, 1662.
4. Fibiger J. Om Serumbehandling af Difteri. *Hospitalstidende* 1898;6;309-25,337-50
5. Hrobjartsson A, Gotzsche P, Gluud C. The controlled clinical trial turns 100 years: Fibiger's trial of serum treatment of diphtheria. BMJ 1998;317; 1243-5.
6. Medical Research Council Therapeutic Trials Committee. The serum treatment of lobar pneumonia. *BrMed J* 1934;i;241-5.
7. Medical Research Council Patulin Trials Committee. Clinical trial of patulin in the common cold. *Lancet* 1944;ii;373-4.
8. Amberson JB, McMahon BL, Pinner MA. A clinical trial of sanocrysin in pulmonary tuberculosis. *Amer Rev Tuberc* 1931;24;401-35.
9. RA Fisher. Statistical methods for research workers. 1925.
10. Hill AB. Principles of medical statistics: I. The aim of the statistical method. *Lancet* 1937;I;41-3.
11. Medical Research Council Whooping-Cough Immunization Committee. The prevention of whooping-cough by vaccination. *Br Med J* 1951;i; 1463-71.
12. Medical Research Council. Streptomycin treatment of pulmonary tuberculosis. BMJ 1948;ii;769-82.
13. Schulz KF, Grimes DA. Generation of allocation sequence in randomised trials: chance, not choice. Lancet 2002;359;515-19.
14. Altman DG, Schulz KF, Moher D, Egger M, Davidoff F, et al. The Revised CONSORT statement for reporting randomised trials: explanation and elaboration. Ann Intern Med 2001;134;663-94.
15. Nicolucci A, Grilli R, Alexanian AA, Apolone G, Torri V, Liberati A. Quality, evolution, and clinical implications of randomised controlled trials on the treatment of lung cancer. A lost opportunity for meta-analysis. JAMA 1989;262;2101-7.
16. Sonis J, Joines J. The quality of clinical trials published in the Journal of Family Practice 1974-1991. J Fam Pract 1994;39;225-35.

17. Ah-See KW, Molony NC. A qualitative assessment of randomised controlled trials in otolaryngology. J Laryngol Otol 1998;112;460-3.
18. Altman DG, Dore CJ. Randomisation and baseline comparisons in clinical trials. Lancet 1990;335;149-53.
19. Moher D, Fortin P, Jadad AR, Juni P, Klassen T, Le Lorier J, et al. Completeness of reporting of trials published in languages other than English: implications for conduct and reporting of systematic reviews. Lancet 1996;347;363-6.
20. Schulz KF, Chalmers I, Grimes DA, Altman DG. Assessing the quality of randomisation from reports of controlled trials published in obstetrics and gynecology journals. JAMA 1994;272;125-28.
21. Adetugbo K, Willams H. How well are randomised controlled trials reported in the dermatology literature? Arch Dermatol 2000;136;381-5.
22. Gluud C, Nikolova D. Quality assessment of reports on clinical trials in the Journal of Hepatology. J Hepatol 1998;29;321-7.
23. Schulz KF, Chalmers I, Hayes RJ, Altman DG. Empirical evidence of bias. Dimensions of methodological quality associated with estimates of treatment effects in controlled trials. JAMA 1995;273;408-12.
24. Kjaergard L, Villumsen J, Gluud C. Quality of randomised clinical trials affects estimates of intervention efficacy. In: Abstract for Workshops and Scientific Sessions, 7th International Cochrane Colloquium, Rome, Italy, 1999.
25. Juni P, Altman DG, Egger M. Assessing the quality of controlled clinical trials. BMJ 2001;323;42-6.
26. Gotzsche PC, Olsen O. Is screening for breast cancer with mammography justifiable? Lancet 2000;355;129-34.
27. Schulz KF. Subverting randomisation in controlled trials. JAMA 1995;274;1456-8.
28. Matts JP, Lachin JM. Properties of permuted-block randomisation in clinical trials. Control Clin Trials 1988;9;327-44.
29. Sleight P et al. for the Heart Outcomes Prevention Evaluation (HOPE) Study Investigators. Blood pressure reduction and cardiovascular risk in HOPE study. *Lancet* 2001;358;2130-1.

30. Lindholm LH, Ibsen H, Dahlof B, et al. Cardiovascular morbidity and mortality in patients with diabetes in the Losartan Intervention For Endpoint reduction in hypertension study (LIFE): randomised trial against atenolol. *Lancet* 2002;359;1004-10.
31. Taylor R. Blood pressure and cardiovascular risk in the HOPE study. *Lancet* 2002;359;2117-8.
32. Bloom JM. Losartan for cardiovascular disease in patients with and without diabetes in the LIFE study. *Lancet* 2002;359;2201.
33. Williams DH, Davis CE. Reporting of assignment methods in clinical trials. Control Clin Trials 1994;15;294-8.
34. Schulz KF, Grimes DA. Unequal group sizes in randomised trials: guarding against guessing. Lancet 2002;359;966-70.
35. Moher D, Pham B, Jones A, Cook DJ, Jadad AR, Moher M, et al. Does quality of reports of randomised trials affect estimates of intervention efficacy reported in meta-analyses? Lancet 1998;352;609-13.
36. Schulz KF, Grimes DA. Allocation concealment in randomised trials: defending against deciphering. Lancet 2002;359;614-8.
37. Gotzsche PC. Methodology and overt and hidden bias in reports of 196 double-blind trials of non-steroidal anti-inflammatory drugs in rheumatoid arthritis. Control Clin Trials 1989;10;31-56.
38. Huwiler-Muntener K, Juni P, Junker C, Egger M. Quality of reporting of randomised trials as a measure of methodological quality. JAMA 2002;287;2801-04.
39. Pildal J, Chan A-W, Hrobjartsson A, Forfang E, Alman DG, Gotzsche PC. Comparison of descriptions of allocation concealment in trial protocols the published reports: cohort study. BMJ 2005;330;1049.
40. Hewitt C, Hahn S, Torgerson DJ, Watson J, Bland JM. Adequacy and reporting of allocation concealment: review of recent trials published in four general medical journals. BMJ 2005;330;1057-8.
41. Soares HP, Daniels S, Kumar A, et al. Bad reporting does not mean bad methods for randomised trials: observational study of randomised trials performed by the Radiation Therapy Oncology Group. BMJ 2004;328; 22-4.

42. Balk EM, Bonis PA, Moskowitz H, et al. Correlation of quality measures with estimates of treatment effect in meta-analyses of randomized controlled trials. JAMA 2002;287;2973-82.
43. Als-Nielsen B, Chen W, Gluud LL, et al. Are trial size and reported methodological quality associated with treatment effects? Observational study of 523 randomised trials. 12th International Cochrane Colloquium, Ottawa, Canada, 2004.
44. Egger M, Juni P, Bartlett C, Holenstein F, Sterne J. How important are comprehensive literature searches and assessment of trial quality in systematic reviews? Empirical study. Health Technol Assess 2003;7;1-76.
45. Wood L, Egger M, Gluud LL, et al. Empirical evidence of bias in treatment effect estimates in controlled trials with different interventions and outcomes: meta-epidemiological study. BMJ 2008;336;601-5.
46. Swingler GH, Zwarenstein M. An effectiveness trial of a diagnostic test in a busy outpatients department in a developing country: issues around allocation concealment and envelope randomisation. J Clin Epidemiol 2000;53;702-6.
47. Schulz KF. Unbiased research and the human spirit: the challenges of randomised controlled trials. CMAJ 1995;153;783-86.
48. Schulz KF. Randomised trials, human nature, and reporting guidelines. Lancet 1996;348;596-8.
49. Egger M, Juni P, Bartlett C. Value of flow diagrams in reports of randomised controlled trials. The CONSORT Group. JAMA 2001;285;1996-9.
50. Kjaergard LL, Nikolova D, Gluud C. Randomised clinical trials in Hepatology: predictors of quality. Hepatology 1999;30;1134-8.
51. Hollis S, Cambell F. What is meant by intention to treat analysis? Survey of published randomised controlled trials. BMJ 1999;319;670-4.
52. Schulz KF, Grimes DA, Altman DG, Hayes RJ. Blinding and exclusions after allocation in randomised controlled trials: survey of published parallel group trials in obstetrics and gynaecology. BMJ 1996;312;742-4.
53. Lee YJ, Ellenberg JH, Hirtz DG, Nelson KB. Analysis of clinical trials by treatment actually received: is it really an option? Stat Med 1991;10; 1595-605.

54. Lewis JA, Machin D. Intention to treat – who should use ITT? Editorial Br J Cancer 1993;68;647-50.
55. Kjaergard LL, Villumsen J, Gluud C. Reporting methodologic quality and discrepancies between large and small randomised trials in meta-analyses. Ann Intern Med 2001;135;982-9.
56. Sackett DL, Gent M. Controversy in counting and attributing events in clinical trials. N Eng J Med 1979;301;1410-2.
57. May GS, DeMets DL, Friedman LM, Furberg C, Passamani E. The randomised clinical trial: bias in analysis. Circulation 1981;64;669-73.
58. Fields WS, Maslenikov V, Meyer JS, Hass WK, Remington RD, MacDonald M. Joint study of extracranial arterial occlusion. V. Progress report of prognosis following surgery or nonsurgical treatment for transient cerebral ischemic attacks and cervical carotid artery lesions. JAMA 1970;211;1993-2003.
59. Kemeny MM, Adak S, Gray B, et al. Combined modality treatment for resectable metastatic colorectal carcinoma to the liver: surgical resection of hepatic metastases in combination with continuous infusion of chemotherapy – an intergroup study. J Clin Oncol 2002;20;1499-505.
60. Kjaergard LL, Krogsgaard K, Gluud C. Interferon alpha with or without ribavirin for chronic hepatitis C: systematic review of randomised trials. BMJ 2001;323;1151-5.
61. Cui L, Hung HM, Wang SJ, Tsong Y. Issues related to subgroup analysis in clinical trials. J Biopharm Stat 2002;12;347-58.
62. Rothwell PM. Treating individuals 2: Subgroup analysis in randomised controlled trials: importance, indications, and interpretation. Lancet 2005;365;176-86.
63. Schulz KF, Grimes DA. Blinding in randomised trials: hiding who got what. Lancet 2002;359;696-700.
64. Day SJ, Altman DG. Statistics notes: blinding in clinical trials and other studies. BMJ 2000;321;504.
65. Campbell IA, Lyons E, Prescott RJ. Stopping smoking. Do nicotine chewing gum and postal encouragement add to doctors' advice? Practitioner 1987;231;114-7.

66. Chalmers TC. Effects of ascorbic acid on the common cold. An evaluation of the evidence. Am J Med 1975;58;532-6.
67. Quitkin FM, Rabkin JG, Gerald J, Davis JM, Klein DF. Validity of clinical trials of antidepressants. Am J Psychiatry 2000;157;327-37.
68. Cheng K, Smyth RL, Motley J, O'Hea U, Ashby D. Randomized controlled trials in cystic fibrosis (1966-1997) categorized by time, design and intervention. Pediatr Pulmonol 2000;29;1-7.
69. O'Malley PG, Balden E, Tomkins G, Santoro J, Kroenke K, Jackson JL. Treatment of fibromyalgia with antidepressants: a meta-analysis. J Gen Intern Med 2000;15;659-66.
70. DerSimonian R, Charette LJ, McPeek B, Mosteller F. Reporing on methods in clinical trials. N Eng J Med 1982;306;1332-7.
71. Khan KS, Daya S, Collins JA, Walter SD. Empirical evidence of bias in infertility research: overestimation of treatment effect in crossover trials using pregnancy as the outcome measure. Fertil Steril 1996;65;939-45.
72. Noseworthy JH, Ebers GC, Vandervoort MK, Farquhar RE, Yetisir E, Roberts R. The impact of blinding on the results of a randomised, placebo-controlled multiple sclerosis clinical trial. Neurology 1994;44;16-20.
73. Max MB. Treatment of post-herpetic neuralgia: antidepressants. Ann Neurol 1994;35(Suppl);S50-3.
74. Gotzsche PC. Blinding during data analysis and writing of manuscripts. Control Clin Trials 1996;17;285-90.
75. Schulz KF, Grimes DA. Multiplicity in randomised trials II: subgroup and interim analyses. Lancet 2005;365;1657-61.
76. Assmann SF, Pocock SJ, Enos LE, Kasten LE. Subgroups analysis and other (mis)uses of baseline data in clinical trials. Lancet 2000;355;1064-9.
77. Yusuf S, Wittes J, Probstfield J, Tyroler HA. Analysis and interpretation of treatment effects in subgroups of patients in randomised clinical trials. JAMA 1991;266;93-8.
78. Pocock SJ, Hughes MD, Lee RJ. Statistical problems in the reporting of clinical trials. A survey of three medical journals. N Eng J Med 1987;317;426-32.

79. Furberg CD, Byington RP. What do subgroup analyses reveal about differential response to beta-bocker therapy? The Beta-blocker Heart Attack Trial experience. Circulation 1983;67;98-101.
80. Tannock IF. False positive results in clinical trials: multiple significance tests and the problems of unreported comparisons. J Natl Cancer Inst 1996;88;206-7.
81. Gelber RD, Goldhirsch A. Interpretation of results from subset analyses within overviews of randomised clinical trials. Stat Med 1987;6;371-88.
82. Hahn S, Williamson PR, Hutton L, Garner P, Flynn EV. Assessing the potential for bias in meta-analysis due to selective reporting of subgroup analysis within studies. Stat Med 2000;19;3325-6.
83. Yusuf S, Collins R, Peto R. Why do we need some large, simple randomised trials? Stat Med 1984;3;409-22.
84. Stallones RA. The use and abuse of subgroup analysis in epidemiological research. Prev Med 1987;16;183-94.
85. Pocock SJ, Hughes MD. Estimation issues in clinical trials and overviews. Stat Med 1990;9;657-71.
86. Brookes ST, Whitley E, Peters TJ, Mulheran PA, Egger M, Davey Smith G. Subgroup analyses in randomised controlled trials: quantifying the risks of false-positives and false-negatives. Health Technol Assess 2001;5;1-56.
87. ISIS-2 Collaborative Group. Randomised trial of intravenous streptokinase, oral aspirin, both, or neither among 17,187 cases of suspected acute myocardial infarction: ISIS-2. Lancet 1988;2;349-60.
88. Cohen LJ. An introduction to the philosophy of induction and probability. Oxford University Press. Oxford, 1989.
89. Moher D, Jones A, Lepage L. Use of the CONSORT statement and quality of reports of randomised trials: a comparative before-and-after evaluation. The CONSORT group. JAMA 2001;285;1992-5.
90. Moher D, Schulz KF, Altman DG. The CONSORT statement: revised recommendations for improving the quality of reports of parallel group randomised trials. The CONSORT Group. Ann Intern Med 2001;134; 657-62.

91. Hill CL, LaValley MP, Felson DT. Secular changes in the quality of published randomised clinical trials in rheumatology. Arthritis Rheum 2002;46; 779-84.
92. Rennie D. Guarding the guardians. *JAMA* 1986;256;2391-2.
93. Altman DG. The scandal of poor medical research. *Br Med J* 1994;308; 283-4.
94. Moher D, Schulz KF, Altman DG. The CONSORT statement: revised recommendations for improving the quality of reports of parallel-group randomised trials. *Lancet* 2001;357;1191-94.

V

A Meagre Offering

Strictly speaking, statistical data apply to groups, not to individuals. But clinicians treat individual patients, not groups, collections or populations. There is, therefore, a problem. It's on display every time the results of a large-scale RCT are cited in order to justify the treatment recommended for a patient. In every case, we could legitimately ask whether the findings are applicable to that particular individual.

Medical researchers evade this issue. They focus instead on whether the results of a study may be generalised to the wider population of patients with the same disease. In statistical terms, they argue from the conclusion about a sample to a generalisation about the underlying population. A study is said to have external validity when its conclusions may be generalised. As will be argued, the conditions for external validity are never fully satisfied.

But there's a separate issue. What is the relevance of statistics-based research to an individual? This depends, amongst other things, on the size of the treatment effect. Large-scale RCTs are necessarily associated with very small benefits. While researchers place undue emphasis on the demonstration of statistical significance, it's the size of the treatment effect that matters to patients. This is what influences their decisions to alter their behaviour or to accept treatment. Ultimately, this is what gives the results of research meaning and relevance.

External Validity

If the trial participants comprise a large randomly selected sample from the entire population of patients with a disease, then it may be argued that the results and conclusions apply to similar randomly selected samples in the future. But study participants aren't selected by a random process. Instead, their recruitment is influenced by such factors as the chosen location of the study, the methods of identification of the participants, and the application of selection criteria.

External Validity

The justification for applying the conclusions of a trial to the wider population of patients

Depends on

- Geographical location
- Setting (primary care, secondary care, academic institutions)
- Selection of patients
- Effect of participation in the study

It's inevitable, therefore, that there will be differences between patients included in, and those excluded from, the study. Thus, any claim that the results of the trial may be generalised is invariably open to challenge on the grounds that patients recruited aren't a representative sample of the broader population. There are, though, other factors that affect the external validity, including the setting of the study.[1,2]

Recruitment of patients to RCTs

As has been often emphasized, the vast majority of patients with a particular disease are never entered into a clinical trial. Most studies are performed in hospitals yet, depending on the disease in question, some patients will not consult their general practitioner, some who do so will not be referred to hospital, and only some of those who reach secondary care will be considered eligible. Estimates suggest that less than 1% of patients will be recruited to trials. Thus, from this measure alone, it's highly unlikely that participants will be representative of the broader population of patients with the disease.

Identification of patients with the disease

In the first instance, the organizers of a large clinical trial decide on the geographical location. In most cases, trials are performed in countries in which the drug is to be marketed, typically those with advanced economies and well developed health care systems. This impairs external validity. Why should we expect the results of a RCT performed in Western Europe or the USA to be applicable to the patients in Africa, Asia or South America?

The number of centres – and, for that matter, the number of countries involved – depends on the size of the study sample required by the protocol together with the incidence or prevalence of the disease. Within the specified geographical location, the choice of centres depends on such factors as local expertise, availability of specialised facilities and the interest of potential investigators. It's not surprising, therefore, to find an undue preponderance of teaching hospitals participating in multi-centre RCTs.

Once the centres have been selected, the identification of patients depends on the disease being studied. For example, cases of rheumatoid arthritis or migraine are readily found in outpatients or general practice whereas patients with acute myocardial infarction are admitted to coronary care units. Clearly, the severity of the disease is affected by

Recruiting Patients to RCTs

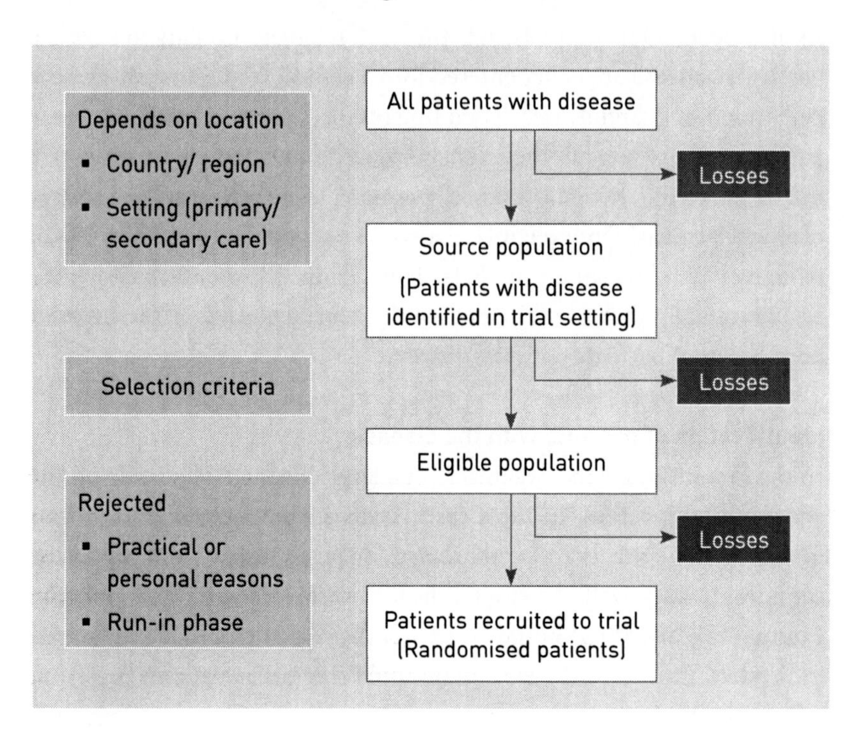

the setting. Depression in general practice, for instance, will tend to be milder than that identified in secondary care. Such differences have important implications for external validity.

Over a specified period of time, a number of patients with the disease will be identified. This group is known as the source population. However, not all of these patients progress further towards recruitment and these losses affect the external validity.[1]

The eligible population

The source population is assessed for eligibility to be included in the trial. This is achieved by applying a set of selection criteria laid down in the protocol. Criteria relate to the characteristics of patients and include age, gender, co-existent medical conditions, current medication, allergies, a history of drug abuse or alcohol dependence, and risk of pregnancy. Admission to the study may require the demonstration of normal laboratory investigations to exclude, for example, renal or hepatic dysfunction. The criteria also relate to the disease being studied. Here, characteristics refer to the severity of the disease, the presence of complications and previous medical or surgical treatment.

The number of selection criteria that contribute to the definition of the eligible population is often large and evidence suggests that it has increased over time.[3] However, due to inadequate reporting, it's often difficult to ascertain the exact criteria used in a RCT and this may seriously limit understanding of how the study participants differ from the general population of patients with the disease.[4,5] But even when selection criteria are included in the publication, their description may be imprecise or vague, allowing considerable scope for interpretation and precluding any firm conclusions as to which patients the results apply.[6-11]

What is clear, however, is that a large proportion of patients in the source population are excluded from clinical trials by the application of selection criteria.[6,11,12,13]

Losses from the eligible population

Not all patients in the eligible population are recruited to the study.[1] The proportion excluded before randomisation is variable and, once again, failure to report accurately the difference between the eligible population and those who were randomised restricts interpretation.[5] There is, however, evidence that losses may be substantial,[14,15] although the reasons are not always apparent. Some eligible patients may become too ill before randomisation, some may develop new medical problems, some may move away from the area, and others may decide not to participate. In many cases, though, there's no readily available explanation.

Perhaps the most obvious example of pruning of the eligible population before randomisation is observed in trials that incorporate a “run-in” phase. This involves giving patients either the active drug or placebo – or each in sequence – before a decision is reached regarding which are to be recruited. Run-in phases are rightly viewed with suspicion, in particular, because of their effect on external validity.[16-18]

A trial that uses a run-in phase with placebo provides information about compliance with medication and allows investigators to exclude patients who would be unlikely take the prescribed treatment according to the protocol. In such circumstances, the results can’t be generalised to the wider population which inevitably includes patients with poor compliance. More importantly, run-in phases that use the active drug provide data not only about compliance but also about both the efficacy and side-effects of medication. This gives the investigators the opportunity to include in the trial only those patients who are likely to comply with treatment, who are known to benefit from the active drug and who are less likely to develop adverse drug reactions – all features that will show the drug in the best possible light but, at the same time, pose a threat to external validity.

A prime example of the potential problems arising from run-in phases may be observed in the HOPE study.[19] This was a large, multi-centre RCT investigating the effect of ramipril – an angiotensin converting enzyme inhibitor – on the prevention of cardiovascular events. Following a run-in phase using active drug and placebo, 10% of 10,576 eligible patients were excluded from randomisation. The reasons for exclusion – which included poor compliance with medication and side-effects such as impaired renal function and hyperkalaemia – were more likely to have been related to ramipril than placebo. The results of the trial were hardly impressive: after five years of treatment, the absolute difference between ramipril and placebo in the primary end-point (a composite of myocardial infarction, stroke or death from cardiovascular disease) was 3.8% while that for overall mortality was 1.8%. Thus, even in the favourable environment created by the run-in phase, only meagre benefits were observed. But what are we to make of the external validity of this study? It can't be argued that the small absolute differences are applicable to the broad population of patients given that 10% of the eligible population were omitted from the trial for reasons related to the outcome. And it's surely also reasonable to suppose that the results of the ramipril group would have been closer to those of the placebo group if the former had included those likely to have developed adverse drug reactions.

This point is well supported by evidence from the carvedilol studies in patients with heart failure.[20, 21] Approximately 5-10% of the eligible population were excluded from randomisation because of an increase in the severity of cardiac failure or the occurrence of adverse drug reactions during the run-in phase. Later it was shown that the occurrence of these two problems in patients receiving carvedilol was less in the randomised trials than it had been in the run-in phases with the drug.

An extreme type of manipulation of the eligible population is observed in trials which preferentially randomise those patients who are already known to benefit from the active drug.[22,23] For example, in a multi-centre RCT of tacrine, a cholinesterase inhibitor used in Alzheimer's disease, only patients who responded to the drug during the run-in phase were randomised.[24] As a result, two-thirds of the eligible population were excluded. In this case, the effect of the run-in phase severely threatens the external validity of the study.

Differences between participants and those excluded from RCTs

Given that those participating in randomised trials are not selected randomly from the population of patients with the particular disease, it's only to be expected that there will be differences between those included in, and those excluded from, RCTs. Such differences have been reported in terms of both demographic and disease-related characteristics.[25-30]

These differences are reflected in the outcomes. Patients excluded from trials tend to have a worse prognosis than those who are recruited.[13,28,31-33] For example, in a large clinical trial of treatment in acute myocardial infarction, the mortality in patients who were excluded from the study was twice that of those who were randomised.[13] These results were supported by a further study in two district general hospitals that participated in thrombolysis trials;[32] only 21% of the source population was actually recruited to the RCTs and the mortality in those included in the trials was 8% compared with 18% in those who were excluded.

These findings confirm that the exclusion of patients from large RCTs affects the external validity.

The environment of a clinical trial

It's not only the differences between the trial participants and the wider population of patients that affect the external validity of RCTs. Other factors related to the environment in which the study is performed are also relevant.

Countries differ in their health care systems – the standards of care, the availability of resources including diagnostic and therapeutic interventions, the standard therapies for diseases and the nature of co-existent illnesses, to name but a few. But, even within the same country, differences exist between the type of institutions which do, and those which do not, participate in RCTs.

Most clinical research is carried out in teaching hospitals by medical staff with both a particular interest in the disease and considerable expertise, supported by nurses with specialist skills and well qualified junior doctors. Under these circumstances, the standard of care would be expected to be high and certainly superior to that of the average district general hospital.[2,34,35] Needless to say, applying the results of RCTs performed in secondary care to patients in general practice, and vice versa, should be done with caution.[36]

The effect of participation in the trial

In addition, participation in a RCT itself may affect the outcome of patients. The close monitoring and requirement to complete the patient record books accurately encourage adherence to the protocol. This includes compliance with treatment regimens, prompt response to the development of new symptoms as well as the early detection and management of complications. Once again, it's unlikely that these circumstances would be present in routine medical practice.

The intractable problem of external validity

It's somewhat ironic that one of the most frequent criticisms of RCTs concerns the failure of external validity.[33,37,38] Randomisation is taken to be a pre-requisite for internal validity and any thought of designing a clinical trial without it would be anathema to researchers. Yet, at the same time, they blithely accept the situation in which randomisation plays no part in the selection of participants to these studies. For those who cherish the statistical foundations of medical research, it must be particularly galling. After all, it's a basic tenet of statistical theory that any inference is dependent on the sample being selected randomly from the underlying population. But, of course, in clinical trials, this condition is never satisfied.

External validity is always going to be under suspicion. Whether it's because of differences between the study participants and the general population of patients with the disease or because of the particular circumstances of the trial, the applicability of the results and conclusions is inevitably going to be open to question.

There is, though, another aspect of clinical trials that must be taken into account when considering external validity. This concerns the very small size of the treatment effect commonly observed in large-scale

RCTs. Relatively small differences between the participants and the wider population may threaten any generalisation of the results.

The failure of external validity is a commonly reported feature of RCTs [14,25,28,29,39-41] and, as has been argued elsewhere,[42-45] it may be responsible for the unwillingness of some medical practitioners to comply with clinical guidelines. But there's little to suggest that it has assumed sufficient importance to stir the medical profession into action. On the contrary, the problem is generally neglected, as emphasized by Rothwell in a thorough account of external validity.[2] Medical researchers, regulatory authorities, ethics committees, journals and the pharmaceutical industry mostly ignore it, preferring instead to concentrate on internal validity.

Perhaps the reluctance to become involved is related to an awareness that, given the current approach to medical research, there's little prospect of improving the situation. Proposed solutions to the problem fare little better. The use of subgroup analysis to identify treatment effects in specific types of patients is, as already discussed, the source of much dispute. For the foreseeable future, flawed external validity is here to stay.

The Meaning of Results of RCTs to Individuals

What do the results of RCTs and epidemiological studies mean to an individual patient? Put another way, what's their relevance and importance? There's no straightforward answer. It depends, for example, on the disease – in particular, the symptoms and the prognosis. A patient who is suffering from intractable pain will attribute importance to the smallest of benefits; on the other hand, someone found to have mild asymptomatic hypertension will need convincing before agreeing to take long-term treatment. It depends on the individual patient – their views about illness and taking medicines, their customs and beliefs. It depends, too, on the end-point of the study. Clinical end-points – especially when they concern serious events – would obviously be considered to be of much greater importance than changes in laboratory measurements. And it depends on the size of the treatment effect.

Meaning of Results to Individual Patients

Depends on

- Symptoms/prognosis of disease
- Attitudes, beliefs, customs
- End-points of study
- Size of treatment effect

In recent times, much has been made of concordance – that is, the practice of providing patients with adequate information so that they may be involved in decisions about their management. But nothing has been done to address the issue of whether the results of large-scale studies on which so many therapeutic decisions are based have any relevance, meaning or importance to individual patients.

The nature of end-points in clinical trials

Although it would be reasonable to expect that the primary end-point of any clinical trial would be that which is of most relevance to patients, this is often not the case. For a disease that may result in the death of some patients, it seems obvious that this would be of major concern. Yet, in many trials in which mortality is relevant, it's not the primary end-point. Instead, less important outcomes are selected on the grounds that the number of deaths in the study participants would be insufficient to demonstrate any statistically significant benefit. And even when mortality is the end-point of a study, it's often restricted to deaths from the disease under investigation – that is, disease-specific mortality, such as deaths from cardiovascular disease or deaths due to colorectal cancer – rather than overall mortality. But are we really to believe that patients are more concerned about the cause of death than that it occurs?

There are, though, specific issues concerning the nature of end-points used in clinical trials that have surfaced in recent years.

Complex measures of disease outcome

If a disease has a single symptom and doesn't progress to complications, then the selection of the end-point is straightforward. The alleviation of the symptom is the appropriate measure of therapeutic success. But most diseases have multiple symptoms and clinical signs, many have laboratory and radiological abnormalities, and often there are demonstrable disturbances in physiological tests. In consequence, it's not uncommon for end-points to incorporate information from a variety of different sources. A good example is observed in clinical trials of treatment in Crohn's disease.[46] In this case, the outcome measure commonly used is the Crohn's disease activity index (CDAI), a numerical score derived from clinical and laboratory data including symptoms – for example, diarrhoea or abdominal pain – findings on examination, measures of nutrition and abnormal investigations such as anaemia, raised inflammatory markers and low blood albumin. Although large reductions in the CDAI usually correlate with clinical improvement, exceptions are not uncommon. Moreover, it's not easy for patients to understand the value of the index when the results clash with their subjective judgement of the efficacy of treatment.

The effect of treatment on many diseases is assessed using complex scales, as observed, for example, in psychiatry and rheumatology[47,48] but, again, the clinical relevance and meaning of such measures is unclear.

Surrogate end-points

It's understandable that investigators are tempted to conduct trials with non-clinical end-points. Changes in biochemical or haematological parameters, physiological measurements or radiological appearances all provide seemingly "objective" endpoints by which to judge the success of treatment. But they're often only loosely connected with clinical outcomes and, in many cases, have been shown to be entirely divorced from what is important and relevant to patients.

Rothwell has described many instances of treatments which, according to surrogate end-points, were shown to be of benefit but which were subsequently demonstrated to have little clinical value.[2] A well known example of this phenomenon relates to the trials of anti-arrhythmic therapy in patients following acute myocardial infarction.[49,50] When judged by a reduction in ectopic beats and arrhythmias on ECG recordings, the drugs were believed to be effective but later studies showed that they failed to improve the clinical outcome – in fact, they were associated with increased mortality. Similarly, reports that beta-interferon was of benefit in multiple sclerosis were based on improvement in the lesions on magnetic resonance imaging but the drug made little difference to the neurological function of patients.[2]

Surrogate endpoints continue to be used in medical research. Over the last decade, the efficacy of drugs for the prevention of osteoporosis has been assessed by changes in bone density. Although treatment has been reported to show an increase in density, this hasn't always been translated into reductions in clinically important outcomes, in particular, fractures of the vertebral column and limb bones.

Surrogate end-points are open to manipulation by pharmaceutical companies keen to promote their products. But, more importantly, they are an obstacle to understanding the meaning and relevance of the results of clinical trials.

Composite end-points

It has become increasingly common for clinical trials to use composite end-points as the primary measure of the efficacy of treatment. On the surface, this appears a useful approach. After all, if patients have ischaemic heart disease, they'll not only want to survive but also to avoid myocardial infarction, cardiac failure, future surgery and admissions to hospital as well as many other problems that they may encounter in the course of their illness. Thus, combining some or all of these features into a "composite" end-point seems reasonable. This, though, isn't the reason why these end-points are used. They are chosen because, by increasing the number of different events that may signal the occurrence of the outcome, they increase the chance of detecting a statistically significant difference in the trial.

But composite end-points are misleading. They combine together events of very different severities and, hence, of difference importance to patients. Moreover, the composite end-point will depend disproportionately on the least clinically important outcome because this usually occurs more frequently – it is, after all, the reason for including events of lesser importance. This leads to misinterpretation on the part of patients and doctors alike. It's easy to assume that a treatment found to reduce a composite end-point which includes mortality will reduce their chances of dying if they take the medication. But composite end-points are disjunctions – not conjunctions – of events and it's a fallacy to infer from a reduction in the composite end-point to a reduction in any one of its component parts.

Of course, the advocates of composite end-points would claim that the individual components are analysed separately as secondary end-points and that the data obtained often show the effect of treatment on individual events. However, as already discussed in the context of subgroup analysis, this leads to further problems.

The size of treatment effects in clinical trials

The decision to recruit large numbers of patients to a RCT reflects the investigators' expectation that the treatment effect will be small. But what's the importance or relevance of such small treatment effects to individual patients? Do patients really understand them? The meaning of a small difference to a particular patient is far from being straightforward.[11]

The relative risk deception

The way in which data from clinical trials are presented is crucial to the understanding of the benefits of treatment. It affects whether doctors prescribe medication and whether patients accept it. The common currency for the effectiveness of treatment in publications of RCTs – and, for that matter, in epidemiological studies – is the relative risk. Yet, it has been recognised for many years that this measure of efficacy is unsuitable because it greatly exaggerates the treatment effect and is, therefore, misleading.[11,51,52]

Consider a simple example of a RCT that shows a mortality of 5% in the placebo group compared with 4% in patients receiving the active drug. The relative risk reduction in mortality is the ratio of the difference in the outcome rates between the placebo and active treatment groups divided by the rate in the placebo group. Hence, in this case, the relative risk reduction is 20%. But this measure of efficacy only applies to patients who would have died if they hadn't received the drug. In other words, the relative risk reduction only refers to a small subgroup of the study participants. This, though, is rarely made clear and, instead, the impression is given that the reduction in outcome applies to all patients given treatment.

Relative Risk Reduction

	Number of patients	Number with outcome	Rate of outcome
Placebo	n_1	x_1	x_1/n_1
Drug	n_2	x_2	x_2/n_2

$$\text{Relative Risk Reduction} = \frac{x_1/n_1 - x_2/n_2}{x_1/n_1}$$

A more accurate measure of efficacy is the absolute risk reduction which is the difference between the mortality rate in the placebo group and that in the active treatment group. In the above example, this amounts to just 1% and, hence, the use of the relative risk reduction yields an estimate of the efficacy of the treatment that is twenty times greater than the absolute difference.

Relative risks are popular with investigators because they make it appear that their work is of more importance than is actually the case. They're also liked by the sponsors of RCTs who use the inflated measures to promote their products. Regrettably, the deception works. Relative risks lead to a favourable interpretation of the results of clinical trials. Compared with absolute risk reductions, they're more likely to persuade doctors – whether in primary or secondary care – to prescribe treatment,[51,53-56] health service managers to pay for drugs [57] and patients to accept medication.[58] Patients, it seems, are impressed by relative risks because many assume that the underlying risk of the unwanted outcome is 100%.[58]

Absolute risk reductions

Small absolute risk reductions are the cardinal feature of large-scale epidemiological studies and RCTs. As the size of clinical trials has increased over recent decades, so the absolute risk reductions have become smaller.[59] Accordingly, many of the drugs used nowadays benefit only a small proportion of patients being treated. For example, in the frequently cited studies of statins and angiotensin-converting enzyme inhibitors, the absolute reduction in the primary end-point was 1.2% to 3.8%.[13,19,60,61] In many clinical situations, less than 5% of patients given long-term treatment will derive any benefit whatsoever.

However, the trivial size of the treatment effects is poorly communicated, both to the medical profession and to patients. Doctors, perhaps beguiled by the promotion of clinical trial results based on relative risks, inaccurately estimate the benefits. When questioned about the efficacy of preventive drugs in cardiovascular disease, more than a quarter of primary care physicians and general internists in the USA overestimated the absolute risk reduction of myocardial infarction by a factor of ten compared with that reported in trials.[62]

When the size of the treatment effects are fully explained, there's evidence that doctors, other health care professionals and, most importantly, patients demand much larger benefits than those reported in RCTs.[63-67] For example, Trewby et al.[67] found that more than three-quarters of patients would decline preventive treatment if the benefit was less than 5% over five years. Clearly, the views of doctors and their patients aren't in line with the recommendations contained in clinical guidelines that are frequently based on small absolute risk reductions.[63-65,67,68]

Making decisions on the basis of small treatment effects

It hardly needs saying that most people don't like taking drugs.[63,69-72] There are many reasons for this aversion to medication which, as studies show, include concerns about both the reliability of the information and the relevance of the results to their everyday lives.[73,74] In the context of large-scale RCTs, both of these concerns are fully justified.

Patients aren't informed of the potential flaws in the internal validity of clinical trials, nor are they given any indication of the problems with external validity. They aren't told about the influence of those with a vested interest in the outcome of clinical trials and, understandably, they know nothing of the fundamental problems concerning the statistical approach to causation on which trials are founded. Were they made aware of the defects associated with medical research, they would be rightly sceptical about accepting treatment based on the results of large clinical trials.

Questions about the relevance and meaning of the results of large statistics-based studies, however, raise further important issues. These relate, in particular, to the nature and size of the end-points. It's only to be expected that complex end-points, surrogate end-points and composite end-points present difficulties in understanding although these may be lessened to some extent by further detailed explanation. However, when it comes to the size of the treatment effect, understanding the meaning and relevance of the results presents special challenges.

Attention has been drawn to the discrepancy between statistical significance and clinical significance of results from large-scale RCTs for more than 20 years.[75-81] Statistically significant differences have little bearing on the clinical importance of the results. This is especially true of large studies with small treatment effects. The concept of a "minimal clinically important difference" – the smallest therapeutic effect that would be considered to justify treatment, taking into account side-effects, inconvenience and cost – was introduced in order to draw attention to this problem.[75-81] Despite its advantages, this approach has been neglected.

Given the problems associated with the interpretation of simple statistical data amongst both the general public and the medical profession,[82] it's not easy to create understanding of the measures of therapeutic efficacy. There are techniques that may be used to improve matters – for instance, the use of pictograms and other visual aids – but there remains a fundamental problem. What is the meaning of a small absolute difference? This isn't answered by replacing one mathematical expression with another – for example, substituting 4 in 100 or 1 in 25 for 4%. The question concerns the meaning of a particular reduction in absolute risk in the context of an individual patient's life.

Imagine someone being informed that his risk of myocardial infarction over the following five years is 7%. How are we to gauge his attitude to this news? Presumably, we do so by his reaction – by what he says and what he does. He may, for instance, express horror, react with utter indifference or look relieved. But whatever his response, it's reasonable to ask whether he would have behaved any differently if he had been told instead that his risk was 6%. It's very difficult to believe that the response would have been any different. And, if this is the case, why should he accept treatment that reduces the risk from 8% to 7%?

Of course, the answer seems obvious: the patient is accepting treatment on the basis of a *reduction* in risk. On closer inspection, though, this is unsatisfactory. Would he accept treatment based on a reduction in risk of any size – for instance, from 0.7% to 0.6% or even from 0.07% to 0.06%? Would we really regard anyone agreeing to continuous medication for five years in order to reduce his risk of myocardial infarction by 1 in 10,000 as behaving sensibly? Surely it's not a matter of *any* reduction in risk but of the size of the reduction. But here, once again, we are brought back to absolute values with their inherent problems of meaning.

Alternatively, the meaning may be sought in personal experiences. Consider again the above example of a drug that reduces mortality from 5% to 4%. What evidence might be available to a patient that would assist in understanding the meaning of this small difference? He may know someone with a similar condition to his own who remained well for five years while taking the medication but he couldn't, of course, infer from this observation that the outcome was due to the drug. Without any treatment, 95% of such patients would be alive while only 1% would have survived because of the medication. There would no single observation that would justify the claim that a particular patient had survived as a result of taking the drug. On the contrary, it would be much more likely that this observation represented an instance of the patient remaining well regardless of the medication. But, were he to hear of a neighbour dying from the disease in question while taking medication, this would be an instance of treatment failure. Thus, the statistical approach to medical research leads to the strange situation in which we can, in the case of individual patients, observe treatment failure but never observe treatment success.

Perhaps, then, he might observe multiple instances in a collection of patients. This would also be of no help. The number needed to show the effect would be the same as that recruited to a large-scale RCT. How is any individual to observe tens of thousands of patients? The point is that there's nothing in an individual's experience that can help him to grasp the meaning of small differences.

The problem of understanding small differences isn't something that we're used to. We don't encounter difficulties with them in the normal course of our lives. We may, for example, want a piece of wood to fit into a space one metre long but we make a mistake and cut a length measuring 101cm. Here, we know what the difference of 1% means: the longer piece won't fit. Or, we may be offered a choice between two savings accounts with different rates of interest, 5% and 4%. Again we know what the 1% difference means: if we choose the first option, we will earn £10 more for every £1,000 invested. But these examples aren't to do with causal phenomena. They concern logic and the effect of the difference is not only certain but also directly observable.

Faced with small differences derived from large-scale RCTs, we don't know what to make of them. It's tempting to think of them in much the same way as we think of the differences between the lengths of wood or the interest rates. But this doesn't work. The meaning of small differences in outcome remains obscure.

Conclusions

The issue of generalising the results of epidemiological studies or large-scale RCTs is an intractable problem facing statistical research. The frequentist approach to statistics entails that the conclusions apply to groups not individuals. This is a considerable drawback in the field of medicine. However, even if we confine any generalisation to groups as opposed to individuals, external validity is always threatened by the failure to select the study sample randomly from the underlying population and by the use of selection criteria. When it comes to statistics-based research, external validity remains an insuperable problem.

Of even greater importance, however, is the question of the value of the product from large-scale RCTs. That the treatment effect is small, is undeniable. But when we look into the matter, it's unclear whether such small absolute differences in outcome between the groups have any meaning or relevance whatsoever to individual patients.

The exaggerated claims in research publications and in the promotional material distributed by pharmaceutical companies have little substance. We can't be sure to whom the results of any large-scale RCT apply and the size of the supposed benefit is trivial. We can't even be certain that it has any meaning whatsoever. For an individual patient, the recommendation to accept treatment on the grounds of the results of statistics-based research is rather like finding a parcel on the doorstep without any name or address on it and which, when opened, is found to be empty. The product of modern-day medical research is very disappointing. So much for the promises made in the early post-war years.

References

1. Elwood JM. Causal relationships in medicine. Oxford University Press. Oxford, England. 1988.
2. Rothwell PM. Treating individuals 1: External validity of randomised controlled trials: "To whom do the results of this trial apply?" Lancet 2005;365;82-93.
3. Fuks A, Weijer C, Freedman B, Shapiro S, Skrutkowska M, Riaz A. A study in contrasts: eligibility criteria in a twenty-year sample of NSABP and POG clinical trials. National Surgical Adjuvant Breast and Bowel Program. Pediatric Oncology Group. J Clin Epidemiol 1998;51;69-79.
4. Hall JC, Mills B, Nguyen H, Hall JL. Methodologic standards in surgical trials. Surgery 1996;119;466-72.
5. Shapiro SH, Weijer C, Freedman B. Reporting the study populations of clinical trials. Clear transmission or static on the line? J Clin Epidemiol 2000;53;973-9.

6. Wilcox RG, et al for the ASSET study group. Trial of tissue plasminogen activator for mortality reduction in acute myocardial infarction. Anglo-Scandinavian Study of Early Thrombolysis (ASSET). *Lancet* 1988;ii;525-30.
7. ISIS-2 (Second International Study of Infarct Survival) Collaborative Group. Randomised trial of intravenous streptokinase, oral aspirin, both or neither among 17187 cases of suspected acute myocardial infarction: ISIS-2. *Lancet* 1988;2;349-60.
8. ISIS-3 (Third International Study of Infarct Survival) Collaborative Group. ISIS-3: a randomised comparison of streptokinase vs tissue plasminogen activator vs anistreplase and of aspirin plus heparin vs aspirin alone among 41,299 cases of suspected acute myocardial infarction. *Lancet* 1992;339; 753-70.
9. LATE Study Group. Late assessment of thrombolytic efficacy (LATE) study with alteplase 6-24 hours after onset of acute myocardial infarction. *Lancet* 1993;342;759-66.
10. Assessment of the Safety and Efficacy of a New Thrombolytic (ASSENT-2) Investigators. Single-bolus tenecteplase compared with front-loaded alteplase in acute myocardial infarction: the ASSENT-2 double-blind randomised trial. *Lancet* 1999;354;716-22.
11. Penston, J. Fiction and fantasy in medical research. The London Press. London, 2003.
12. Gruppo Italiano per lo Studio della Sopravvivenza nell'Infarcto Miocardico. GISSI-2: a factorial randomised trial of alteplase versus streptokinase and heparin versus no heparin among 12,490 patients with acute myocardial infarction. *Lancet* 1990;336;65-71.
13. Gruppo Italiano per lo Studio della Sopravvivenza nell'Infarcto Miocardico. GISSI-3: effects of lisinopril and transdermal glyceryl trinitrate singly and together on 6-week mortality and ventricular function after acute myocardial infarction. *Lancet* 1994;343;1115-22.
14. Gilbody S, Wahlbeck K, Adams C. Randomised controlled trials in schizophrenia: a critical perspective on the literature. Acta Psychiatr Scand 2002;105;243-51.

15. Muller DW, Topol EJ. Selection of patients with acute myocardial infarction for thrombolytic therapy. Ann Intern Med 1990;113;949-60.
16. Haynes RB, Dantes R. Patient compliance and the conduct and interpretation of therapeutic trials. Control Clin Trials 1987;8;12-9.
17. Gomez-Marin O, Prineas RJ, Sinaiko AR. The sodium-potassium blood pressure trial in children: design, recruitment and randomisation. Control Clin Trials 1991;12;408-23.
18. Pablos-Mendez A, Barr RG, Shea S. Run-in periods in randomised trials: implications for the application of results in clinical practice. JAMA 1998;279;222-5.
19. Yusuf S, et al. for the Heart Outcomes Prevention Evaluation Study Investigators. Effects of an angiotensin-converting-enzyme inhibitor, ramipril, on cardiovascular events in high-risk patients. *New Eng J Med* 2000;342;145-153.
20. Australia-New Zealand Heart Failure Research Collaborative Group. Effects of carvedilol, a vasodilatory β-blocker, in patients with congestive heart failure due to ischaemic heart disease. Circulation 1995;92; 212-8.
21. Packer M, Bristow MR, Cohn JN, et al. The effects of carvedilol on morbidity and mortality in patients with chronic heart failure. US Carvedilol Heart Failure Study group. N Eng J Med 1996;334;1349-55.
22. Hallstrom AP, Verter J, Friedman L. Randomising responders. Control Clin Trials 1991;12;486-503.
23. Leber PD, Davis CS. Threats to the validity of clinical trials employing enrichment strategies for sample selection. Control Clin Trials 1998;19; 178-87.
24. Davis KL, Thai LJ, Gamzu ER, et al. The Tacrine Collaborative Study Group. A double-blind, placebo-controlled multicenter study of tacrine for Alzheimer's disease. N Eng J Med 1992;327;1253-9.
25. Licht RW, Gouliaev G, Vestergaard P, Frydenberg M. Generalisability of results of randomised drug trials. Br J Psychiatry 1997;170;264-67.
26. Gurwitz JH, Col NF, Avorn J. The exclusion of elderly and women from clinical trials in acute myocardial infarction. JAMA 1992;268;1417-22.

27. Bjorn M, Brendstrup C, Karlsen S, Carlsen JE. Consecutive screening and enrolment in clinical trials: the way to representative patient samples? J Card Fail 1998;4;225-30.
28. Brown N, Melville M, Gray D, et al. Relevance of clinical trial results in myocardial infarction to medical practice: comparison of four year outome in participants of a thrombolytic trial, patients receiving routine thrombolysis, and those deemed ineligible for thrombolysis. Heart 1999;81;598-602.
29. Britton A, McKee M, Black N, McPherson K, Sanderson C, Bain C. Threats to applicability of randomised trials: exclusions and selective participation. J Health Serv Res Policy 1999;4;112-21.
30. Moore DA, Goodall RL, Ives NJ, Hooker M, Gazzard BG, Easterbrook PJ. How generalisable are the results of large randomised controlled trials of antiretroviral therapy? HIV Med 2000;1;149-54.
31. Woods KI, Ketley D, Ludman PF, et al. Intravenous beta blockade in acute myocardial infarction. Doubt exists about external validity of trials of intravenous beta blockade. BMJ 1999;318;328-9.
32. Dixon G, Boyle RM, Norris RM. Clinical trials in acute myocardial infarction versus real life: a limitation of evidence-based medicine. *Br J Cardiol* 2000;7;709-11.
33. Hampton JR. Size isn't everything. Stat Med 2002;21;2807-14.
34. Downs SH, Black NA, Devlin HB, Royston CM, Russell RC. Systematic review of the effectiveness and safety of laparascopic cholecystectomy. Ann R Coll Surg Eng 1996;78;241-323.
35. Roberts C. The implications of variation in outcome between health professionals for the design and analysis of randomised controlled trials. Stat Med 1999;18;2605-15.
36. Mant D. Can randomised trials inform clinical decisions about individual patients? Lancet 1999;353;743-6.
37. Charlton BG, Miles A. The rise and fall of EBM. Q J Med 1998;91;371-74.
38. Feinstein AR, Horwitz RI. Problems in the "evidence" of "evidence-based medicine". Am J Me 1997;103;529-35.
39. Benech I, Wilson AE, Dowell AC. Evidence-based practice in primary care: past, present and future. J Eval Clin Pract 1996;2;249-63.

40. Egglin TK, Horwitz RI. The case for better research standards in peripheral thrombolysis: poor quality of randomised trials during the past decade. Acad Radiol 1996;3;1-9.
41. Norris SL, Engelgau MM, Narayan KM, Effectiveness of self management training in type 2 diabetes: a systematic review of randomised controlled trials. Diabetes Care 2001;24;561-87.
42. Fahey T. Applying the results of clinical trials to patients in general practice: perceived problems, strengths, assumptions, and challenges for the future. Br J Gen Pract 1998;48;1173-8.
43. Pashos CL, Normand SL, Garfinkle JB, Newhouse JP, Epstein AM, McNeil BJ. Trends in use of drug therapies in patients with acute myocardial infarction: 1988 to 1992. J Am Coll Cardiol 1994;23;1023-30.
44. Grol R, Dalhuijsen J, Thomas S, et al. Attributes of clinical guidelines that influence use of guidelines in general practice: observational study. BMJ 1998;317;858-61.
45. Sonis J, Doukas D, Klinkman M, Reed B, Ruffin MT. Applicability of clinical trial results to primary care. J Am Med Assoc 1998;280;1746.
46. Best WR, Becktel JM, Singleton JW, Kern F. Development of a Crohn's disease activity index. National Copoperative Crohn's Disease Study. Gastroenterology 1976;70;439-44.
47. Gotzsche PC. Methodology and overt and hidden bias in reports of 196 double-blind trials of non-steroidal anti-inflammatory drugs in rheumatoid arthritis. Control Clin Trials 1989;10;31-56.
48. Thornley B, Adams C. Content and quality of 2000 controlled trials in schizophrenia over 50 years. BMJ 1998;317;1181-4.
49. McAlistair FA, Teo KK. Antiarrhythmic therapies for the prevention of sudden cardiac death. Drugs 1997;54;235-52.
50. The Cardiac Arrhythmia Suppression Trial (CAST) Investigators. Preliminary report: effect of encainide and flecainide on mortality in a randomised trial of arrhythmia suppression after myocardial infarction. N Eng J Med 1989;321;406-12.

51. Naylor CD, Chen E, Strauss B. Measured enthusiasm: does the method of reporting trial results alter perceptions of therapeutic effectiveness? Ann Intern Med 1992;117;916-21.
52. Skolbekken J-A. Communicating the risk reduction achieved by cholesterol reducing drugs. BMJ 1998;316;1956-8.
53. Forrow L, Taylor WC, Arnold RM. Absolutely relative: how research results are summarized can affect treatment decisions. Am J Med 1992;92;121-4.
54. Bobbio M, Demichelis B, Giustetto G. Completeness of reporting trial results: effect on physicians' willingness to prescribe. Lancet 1994;343;1209-11.
55. Bucher HC, Weinbacher M, Gyr K. Influence of method of reporting study results on decisions of physicians to prescribe drugs to lower cholesterol concentrations. BMJ 1994;309;761-4.
56. Cranney M, Walley T. Same information, different decisions: the influence of evidence on the management of hypertension in the elderly. Br J Gen Pract 1996;46;661-3.
57. Fahey T, Griffiths S, Peters TJ. Evidence based purchasing: understanding results of clinical trials and systematic reviews. BMJ 1995;311;1056-9.
58. Malenka DJ, Baron JA, Johansen S, Wahrenberger JW, Ross JM. The framing effect of relative and absolute risk. J Gen Intern Med 1993;8;543-8.
59. Freemantle N & Hill S. Medicalisation, limits to medicine, or never enough money to go around? *Br Med J* 2002;324;864-5.
60. The Long-Term Intervention with Pravastatin in Ischaemic Disease (LIPID) Study Group. Prevention of cardiovascular events and death with pravastatin in patients with coronary heart disease and a broad range of initial cholesterol levels. *New Eng J Med* 1998;339;1349-57.
61. Plehn JF, Davis BR, Sacks FM, et al. Reduction of stroke incidence after myocardial infarction with pravastatin: the Cholesterol and Recurrent Events (CARE) Study. *Circulation* 1999;99;216-23.
62. Friedmann PD, Brett AS, Mayo-Smith MF. Differences in generalists' and cardiologists' perceptions of cardiovascular risk and the outcomes of preventive therapy in cardiovascular disease. Ann Intern Med 1996;124; 414-421.

63. Lewis DK, Robinson J, Wilkinson E. Factors involved in deciding to start preventive treatment: qualitative study of clinicians' and lay people's attitudes. BMJ 2003;327;841.
64. Lewis DK, Barton S. Who decides when to start preventive treatment? A questionnaire survey to compare the views of different population subgroups. J Epidemiol Community Health 2003;57;241-2.
65. Steel N. Thresholds for taking antihypertensive drugs in different professional and lay groups: questionnaire survey. BMJ 2000;320;1446-7.
66. MacAlister FA, O'Connor AM, Wells G, Grover SA, Laupacis A. When should hypertension be treated? The different perspectives of Canadian family physicians and patients. Canadian Medical Association Journal 2000;163;403-8.
67. Trewby PN, Reddy AV, Trewby CS, Ashton VJ, Brennan G, Inglis J. Are preventive drugs preventive enough? A study of patients' expectation of benefit from preventive drugs. Clin Med 2002;2;527-33.
68. Montgomery AA, Harding J, Fahey T. Shared decision making in hypertension: the impact of patient preferences on treatment choice. Family Practice 2001;18;309-13.
69. Donovan JL, Blake DR. Patient non-compliance: deviance or reasoned decision-making. Soc Sci Med 1992;34;507-13.
70. Britten N. Patients' ideas about medicine: a qualitative study in a general practice population. B J Gen Pract 1994;44;465-8.
71. Benson J, Britten N. Patients' decision about whether or not to take antihypertensive drugs. BMJ 2002;325;873-6.
72. Townsend A, Hunt K, Wyke S. Managing multiple morbidity in mid-life: a qualitative study of attitudes to drug use. BMJ 2003;327;837-40.
73. Haynes RB, Devereaux PJ, Guyatt GH. Clinical expertise in the era of evidence-based medicine and patient choice. Evidence-Based Medicine 2002;7;36-8.
74. Alaszewski A, Horlick-Jones T. How can doctors communicate information about risk more effectively? BMJ 2003;327;728-31.
75. Pocock SJ, Hughes MD, Lee RJ. Statistical problems in reporting clinical trials: a survey of three medical journals. N Eng J Med 1987;317;426-32.

76. Wells GA, Tugwell P, Kraag GR, Baker PR, Goh J, Redelmeier DA. Minimum important difference between patients with rheumatoid arthritis: the patients' perspective. Journal of Rheumatology 1993;20;557-60.
77. Moher D, Dulberg CS, Wells GA. Statistical power, sample size and their reporting in randomised controlled trials. JAMA 1994;272;122-4.
78. Guyatt GH, Juniper EF, Walter SD, Griffith LE, Goldstein RS. Interpreting treatment effects in randomised trials. BMJ 1998;316;690-3.
79. Juniper EF. Quality of life questionnaires: does statistically significant = clinically important? Journal of Allergy and Clinical Immunology 1998;102;16-7.
80. Chan KB, Man-Song-Hing M, Molnar FJ, Laupacis A. How well is the clinical importance of study results reported? An assessment of randomised controlled trials. Canadian Medical Association Journal 2001;165;1197-202.
81. Jones PW. Interpreting thresholds for a clinically significant change in health status in asthma and COPD. European Respiratory J 2002;19;398-404.
82. Gigerenzer G. Reckoning with risk. The Penguin Press. London, 2002.

VI

A Squabble of Statisticians

Much rides on the validity of statistical analysis in medical research. Once bias and the unequal distribution of relevant factors have been excluded – as, indeed, they are claimed to be in RCTs – it's left to the statisticians to pass judgment on whether the difference in outcome between the groups is simply due to chance or indicates the presence of a causal relationship.

The dominant branch of statistics is that based on the frequentist theory. This includes Fisher's significance testing and the Neyman-Pearson hypothesis test – or, more commonly nowadays, a hybrid version of the two approaches – and it permeates many diverse academic disciplines from medical research to the social sciences. But is it really as sound as we are led to believe? The medical community, it seems, has few qualms. There's precious little in the way of criticism concerning the fundamental aspects of frequentist theory either in medical journals or in the standard textbooks of statistics used by clinical researchers and medical practitioners.[1]

It will, therefore, be news to many involved in medical research that there's much disquiet about conventional statistical analysis. Trenchant criticism has been aired many times over the past fifty years or more yet this has been mostly confined to specialist statistical texts. On the rare occasions when it does surface in the medical literature, it makes little impact.

Given that most clinical and epidemiological research in recent times has been grounded on the frequentist theory, any recognition that this approach to statistical analysis is seriously flawed would bring into question much of the so-called knowledge that provides the basis of most medical practice today.

The Frequentist Approach

Probability according to frequentist theory

According to the standard textbooks of statistics, particularly those used in medical education, probability would appear to be straightforward. But the various theories of probability [2] and the fundamental philosophical differences between them are seldom touched upon even though they are essential for any genuine understanding of the statistics that arises from them.

The frequentist account of probability is based on the idea of the long-run relative frequency of a characteristic within a reference class. We may, for example, want to know the probability of the original clutch of a Vauxhall Vectra lasting for 50,000 miles. Accordingly, we would make observations on a large number such cars that had travelled 50,000 miles (the reference class) and determine the number that still have the original clutch (the characteristic). The probability we are seeking would be equal to the number of cars with the original clutch divided by the number of cars observed to have travelled 50,000 miles.

For the frequentists, there's nothing more to probability than the relative frequency with which a characteristic occurs in a specified reference class. They believe that these relative frequencies are to be found in countless phenomena in the natural world. From this point of view, probability is something that exists independently of human beings. It has nothing to do with what we think or believe. Instead, probability is considered to be objective.[2-5]

Frequentist Theory of Probability

- Based on the long-run relative frequency

$$\text{Probability of X} = \frac{\text{Number of instances of X}}{\text{Number of instances of reference class}}$$

But...

- It only applies to situations where repeated observations are possible
- It does not apply to individuals

But it's apparent from the start that this approach to probability is unsatisfactory. It clearly only applies to a situation in which there is the possibility of making repeated observations of items from the reference class to determine how often the characteristic occurs. Yet we often make probability statements about circumstances that are not repeatable. We speak, for example, of the probability that Labour will win the next election under a new leader or that Crazy Jack will win in his first Grand National. These are particular situations, the circumstances of which have never been present in the same way in the past. They're not subject to repeated observations. Nonetheless, we do attribute probabilities in these situations. People, for example, place bets on such outcomes. At the very least, we must conclude that the frequentist approach fails to offer a comprehensive account of probability and we may favour, instead, other theories that are applicable to a wider range of circumstances.

Even when the frequentist approach is used in appropriate situations, it has a major drawback. Probabilities based on the relative frequency don't apply to individuals.[2] There is, however, a great temptation to believe the opposite. When we think of probability, our minds often turn to games of chance. This is understandable. History shows that probability arose from games of chance and, indeed, the link persists in modern textbooks where the simple concepts of probability are presented in the terms of the outcomes of dice-throwing and card games. In such cases, probability does apply to individual instances. Games of chance are based on what is known as the indifference theory of probability.[2] Here, the probability of any particular outcome is equal to the number of ways in which that outcome may occur divided by the total number of possible outcomes. Thus, the probability of throwing a three with a fair die is 1/6 and that of throwing an even number is 3/6. Behind the indifference theory is the principle that all outcomes are equally probable if there's no reason why one should occur more or less often than another. But this isn't based on any empirical data. It's a rule of any game of chance. Once this is accepted, it follows that the probabilities apply to all throws of a fair die because *a priori* the conditions are the same.

Such an argument doesn't apply to the frequentist theory. The grounds for claiming that we have no reason to believe in one outcome more than another are missing. On the contrary, we expect there to be differences in outcome amongst individuals. There would, after all, be no point in the frequentist theory unless there was uncertainty and this uncertainty resides in the differences – both known and unknown – between the members of the reference class which relate to differences in the occurrence of the characteristic. It's this heterogeneity that precludes any assertion that what applies to the reference class as a whole applies equally to individual members of that class. A probability statement based on the relative frequency applies only to the reference class collectively.

We may say, for example, that the probability of the clutch surviving 50,000 miles based on the analysis of a large sample is 0.6 but this hardly applies to the Vauxhall Vectra owned by a driving instructor who, day in and day out, witnesses assaults on the clutch of his car. The members of a reference class are anonymous and the probability applies to them collectively. But once an individual member is identified – once we know something about it – the relative frequency can no longer be said to apply.

Thus, the heterogeneity in the reference class that is the reason for developing probability theories is the source of one of the main criticisms of the frequentist approach to statistics. Frequentists pool together members of the reference class and believe that this leads to worthwhile results in their studies. But they can never escape from the problems associated with the fact that they are dealing with mixtures of very different individuals, the precise composition of which they remain in ignorance.

RA Fisher

The origin of the statistical approach that has dominated medical research for more than fifty years may be traced back to the seminal work of RA Fisher in the early 20th century.[6,7] Although he wasn't involved directly with epidemiological or clinical studies, there can be little doubt about his central role in the development of what is now considered to be the orthodox methodology.[8] Fisher, more than anyone else, is responsible for the way in which medical research is carried out today. In textbooks and scientific papers, he provided a detailed account of an entirely new method for the investigation of natural phenomena.

Fisher was primarily a statistician – indeed, given the originality of his contributions to the subject, many consider him to be the foremost statistician of the last century. While working in agricultural research in the years after the First World War, he recognised the difficulties involved in excluding chance as an explanation for the differences in the yield of crops in field trials. In *Statistical Methods for Research Workers*,[6] he described the basics of the frequentist approach to statistics, beginning with the central role of populations.

> "... statistics is the study of populations, or aggregates of individuals, rather than of individuals." [6]

The individuals making up these populations aren't necessarily physical objects; they may, for example, be measurements taken in the course of repeated experiments or even the results of calculations on these measurements. But they always show differences.

> "The populations which are the object of statistical study always display variation in one or more respects." [6]

Take, for example, Cox's Orange Pippins. They vary in terms of their characteristics including colour, shape, size, weight, and taste. If we had all of these apples before us, we may describe their weight using tables or histograms showing the proportion of the population in various classes defined by a range of values. This is the frequency distribution and it is fundamental to Fisher's statistics. Alternatively, the population may be described in terms of constants or parameters. In this case, the relevant parameters would be the mean and variance of the weight of apples. Of course, in most cases, we don't have the entire population available for inspection. Hence, the parameters are unknown.

> "We cannot in fact know the specification exactly, but we can make estimates of the unknown parameters which will be more or less exact. These estimates, which are termed statistics, are of course calculated from the observations." [6]

Random samples drawn from the underlying population provide information about the parameters. If we take a large sample of Cox's Orange Pippins, the mean weight – a statistic – will tend towards the true value of the population mean. But statistics like the mean are random variables with a range of values. A single mean obtained from a random sample is just one of a range of means that would be found in the course of repeated sampling. If we are to use the sample mean to draw inferences, we require a measure of the error associated with that statistic.

Fisher's tests of significance

According to Fisher, the idea behind the test of significance is to...

> "...examine whether or not the data are in harmony with any suggested hypothesis." [6]

The process of investigating natural phenomena begins with a hypothesis. This is a precise statement about a parameter from the underlying population. Data are then collected and the value of the statistic chosen to estimate the parameter is calculated. Finally, the statistic is compared with the distribution of values associated with the hypothesis.

> "For a given population we may calculate the probability with which any sample will occur, and if we can solve the purely mathematical problem presented, we can calculate the probability of occurrence of any given statistic calculated from such a sample." [6]

In other words, the test of significance allows us to judge whether the data observed are due to chance. To shed further light on this, consider a hypothetical large RCT which reported a reduction in mortality from 12% with placebo to 10% with the active drug. How are we to determine whether the difference in mortality of 2% between the two groups is due to chance or, instead, is the result of treatment? The basic assumption underlying the significance test is the truth of the null hypothesis (H_0) which states that there's no difference in the outcome between placebo and the active drug. Put another way, if H_0 is true, the two samples are drawn from the same population.

In this case, the statistic being tested is the difference in outcomes between the two groups. This is just one of a population of differences. If the trial were to be repeated many times, there would be a range of values for the difference assuming H_0 were true. Thus, to determine whether the result is due to chance, we have to compare the value of the statistic with the distribution of differences in the population given H_0. The frequency distribution of the differences becomes the background against which the observed result is to be compared.

> "The idea of an infinite population distributed in a frequency distribution in respect of one or more characters is fundamental to all statistical work. From a limited experience... we may obtain some idea of the infinite hypothetical population from which our sample is drawn, and so of the probable nature of future samples to which our conclusions are to be applied. If a second sample belies this expectation we infer that it is, in the language of statistics, drawn from a different population... Critical tests of this kind may be called tests of significance, and when such tests are available we may discover whether a second sample is or is not significantly different from the first." [6]

The significance test gives a measure of the probability of obtaining a result equal to or more extreme than that observed given the truth of the null hypothesis. This is known as the P-value.

P-value

The probability of obtaining a result equal to or greater than that observed in the study on the assumption that the null hypothesis is true

= Probability [data/truth of null hypothesis]

= $P[d/H_0]$

Low P-values lead to the rejection of H_0. But where is the line to be drawn? In his earlier works, Fisher was clear on the matter.

"The value for which P = 0.05, or 1 in 20, is 1.96 or nearly 2; it is convenient to take this point as a limit in judging whether a deviation is to be considered significant or not. Deviations exceeding twice the standard deviation are thus formally regarded as significant." [6]

Although he recommended that a P-value of 0.05 be accepted as the cut-off level for rejecting H_0, he emphasized that any particular P-value was open to interpretation on the part of researchers. But his willingness to accept a degree of subjectivity into significance testing led him into conflict with those who viewed science as a strictly objective enterprise.

Fisher and the randomised trial

To most researchers, Fisher's importance lies in his development of the randomised trial. They see randomisation solely as a process to deliver groups with an equal distribution of variables relevant to the outcome of the trial. Bradford Hill, for example, recognised this as the crucial role for randomisation as early as the 1930's [9] and this view has persisted.[8]

In contrast, Fisher believed that the primary role of randomisation was to ensure the validity of statistical inference. In order to test whether a difference between two groups is statistically significant, we need estimates of the errors involved. The reliability of these estimates depends on randomisation.

"The error of which an estimate is required is that in the difference in yield between... plots treated differently in respect of the manure tested. The estimate of error afforded by the replicated trial depends upon differences between plots treated alike. An estimate of error so derived will only be valid for its purpose if we make sure that, in the plot arrangement, pairs of plots treated alike are not nearer together, or further apart than, or in any other relevant way, distinguishable from pairs of plots treated differently...

One way of making sure that a valid estimate of error will be obtained is to arrange the plots deliberately at random so that no distinction can creep in between pairs of plots treated alike and pairs treated differently; in such a case an estimate of error... may be applied to test the significance of the observed difference between the averages of plots treated differently." [10]

Fisher's agricultural experiments resemble modern-day RCTs. A field is divided into a large number of plots of equal size and each plot is either left untreated or receives manure depending on random allocation. Each of the two groups of plots provides multiple observations relating to the crop yield. These observations allow the calculation of the difference in crop yield and provide an estimate of the error of this statistic. The observed difference is then compared with the distribution of differences that would be expected if H_0 were true in order to determine whether or not the result is statistically significant.

As Fisher pointed out,[6] valid estimates of the error depend on the differences in background conditions between the two groups being minimised. If the two groups are closely matched, then the error derived from multiple observations in each group will be similar. Thus, randomisation is a fundamental requirement for valid estimates of error and, hence, it is essential for statistical inference.[6-9,11]

Fisher's Solution to the Problem of Heterogeneity

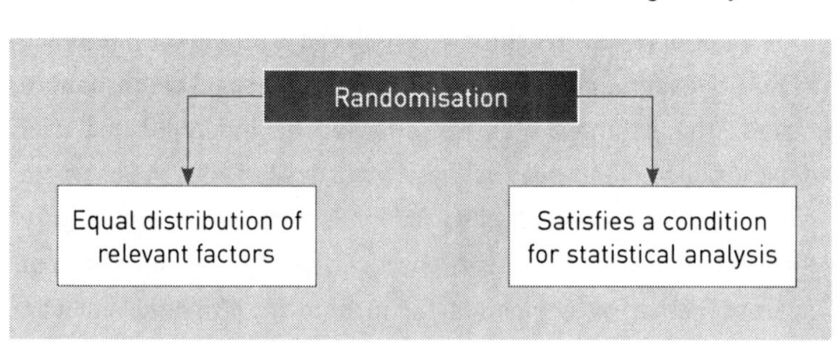

Therefore, randomisation serves two important functions. Firstly, it ensures that factors relevant to the outcome are distributed equally between the two groups, thus satisfying an important condition for internal validity. Secondly, it is a basic requirement for the validity of statistical analysis.

Neyman-Pearson hypothesis testing

As noted above, Fisher wasn't in favour of a rigid interpretation of P-values and preferred investigators to have some latitude. In the 1930's, Neyman and Pearson sought to remove this element of subjectivity and introduced a procedure known as hypothesis testing.[12]

The Neyman-Pearson approach involves two hypotheses: the null hypothesis (H_0) and the alternative hypothesis (H_a), often referred to as the research hypothesis. Before the trial begins, decisions are made concerning the degree of error that is considered acceptable.

Type I error involves the rejection of H_0 when H_0 is true. The probability of a Type I error is known as β. In the course of a long series of similar experiments, if α is set at 0.05, then 5% or less of null hypotheses that are true will be rejected.

Neyman-Pearson Hypothesis Testing

	Do not reject H_0	Reject H_0
H_0 True	Correct	Type I error
H_0 False	Type II error	Correct

Type II error is the failure to reject H_0 when H_0 is false and is known as β. If H_0 and H_a are mutually exclusive, a Type II error also results from the rejection of H_a when H_a is true.

The error rates, α and β, are specified in advance of the study and chosen to minimise the risks of making an incorrect decision between H_o and H_a. As in the case of significance testing, the difference in outcome between the two groups is calculated and compared with the distribution of differences under the null hypothesis. Here, though, the similarities end. Whereas in significance testing the next step is to calculate the P-value, in hypothesis testing it is to determine whether or not the observed result falls within a particular tail area under the distribution curve defined by alpha and known as the rejection region. If the observed difference falls within this area, then H_o is to be rejected.

Hence, there's no decision to be made after the statistical analysis and there's no interpretation. Everything has already been decided before the trial began. The unwanted subjectivity has been eradicated – but, at a cost.

> "... no test based upon a theory of probability can by itself provide any valuable evidence of the truth or falsehood of a hypothesis. But we may look at the purpose of tests from another viewpoint. Without hoping to know whether each separate hypothesis is true or false, we may search for rules to govern our behaviour with regard to them, in following which we insure that, in the long run of experience, we shall not often be wrong." [12]

This passage makes clear the problem that arises. While the Neyman-Pearson procedure offers a way of choosing between two hypotheses, its justification requires a large number of studies over time. But the procedure provides no grounds for inferring causation in an individual study. Neyman and Pearson sacrificed Fisher's significance testing – which supports causal inference – in order to eliminate Fisher's subjectivity.[13]

Criticism of Frequentist Statistics

The widespread use of P-values and hypothesis testing suggests that the medical community has no serious doubts about the statistical methods used in clinical and epidemiological studies. All, it seems, is well. Yet, anyone drawing the conclusion that the frequentist theory is unproblematic would be wrong.

> "It is one of the most disturbing yet poorly-recognised facts of contemporary science that such qualms [about frequentist methods] are far from misplaced. There are indeed fundamental problems with the standard methods of statistical inference and warnings about their impact on scientific research have been repeatedly pointed out for over 30 years in mathematical research papers and even general science publications. So far, however, these warnings have had virtually no effect beyond the community of mathematical statisticians." [14]

There can be little dispute that warnings about the unreliability of the frequentist approach have been repeatedly issued since the 1930s.[1, 13-37] Frequentist statistics has been accused of being confusing and poorly understood by researchers, the charge has been made that it's fundamentally flawed, and it's claimed that it hinders rather than promotes advances in science. It's widely reproached for not addressing what is important and relevant to research. Calls have even been made for its methods to be abandoned.[20,21]

Those involved in research who routinely use statistics based on the frequentist theory – whether in medicine, the social sciences or other disciplines – will react to such remarks with incredulity. But it's not difficult to justify the criticisms.

Criticisms of Frequentist Statistics

"The null hypothesis of no difference has been judged to be no longer a sound or fruitful basis for statistical investigation... Significance tests do not provide the information that scientists need, and, furthermore, they are not the most effective method for analyzing and summarising data." [19]

"... the test of statistical significance in psychological research may be taken as an instance of a kind of essential mindlessness in the conduct of research."[16]

"... a great deal of mischief has been associated with its use." [16]

"... nothing but... pseudo-intellectual garbage."[18]

"... science becomes an automated, blind search for mindless tabular asterisks using thoughtless hypotheses." [37]

"Many researchers believe that statistical significance testing confers important benefits that are in fact completely imaginary." [26]

"Null-hypothesis significance testing is surely the most bone-headedly misguided procedure ever institutionalized in the rote of training of science students." [36]

"... I find it difficult to imagine a less insightful means of transiting from data to conclusions." [35]

"The collective illusions about the meaning of a significant result are embarrassing to our profession." [1]

The troublesome P-value

Does anyone really know what it means?

Whatever the level of education – whether in school, at university or during post-graduate studies – the initial confrontation with the P-value is likely to produce a sense of bewilderment which hardly lessens with the passage of time. How many researchers, let alone qualified doctors or students, are able to give an accurate definition of the P-value? How many really understand it? It seems very few do. But is this because they're particularly stupid? Are their teachers simply incompetent? Or is it rather that there's something fundamentally wrong with P-values?

Gigerenzer has written extensively about the problems involved in understanding numerical and statistical data, with particular regard to conditional probabilities.[1,38] In one study, he investigated the ability of students, lecturers and professors of psychology in Germany to interpret relatively simple statements about the P-value.[1] All of the students and 80% of those lecturers and professors who actually taught the null hypothesis answered at least some of the questions incorrectly. These results were similar to those obtained in the United Kingdom [39] and Israel.[31]

In the light of these findings, it would be easy to blame those involved in teaching statistics for the woeful level of understanding of this fundamental concept. On the other hand, perhaps there's a basic problem with the nature of the P-value.

Getting the wrong end of the stick: mistakes about the P-value

Misunderstandings regarding P-values are common and seem to arise either from neglecting the true definition of the P-value or from logical errors in the interpretation of its meaning. The mistakes and confusions concerning P-values have been meticulously reviewed by Nickerson.[33]

(i) Studies indicate that many people believe that the P-value is the probability of H_0 being true.[4,13,20,27,31,33,40-42] Thus, a P-value of 0.05 is taken to mean that there is a 5% probability that H_0 is true. But, since the P-value is founded on the assumption that H_0 is true, it can't at the same time be used to comment on the whether or not H_0 is true. The fallacy is based on an incorrect understanding of the definition of the P-value.

(ii) Others make the mistake of believing that the P-value is the probability of H_0 given the observed data. This is the error of believing that $P[d/H_0]$ is equal to $P[H_0/d]$. But these two conditional probabilities are not the same.[14,20,33,40,43,44]

Consider, for example, the relationship between the diagnosis that a patient has a myocardial infarction (A) and the observation that the patient has chest pain (B). While most patients who suffer a heart attack complain of chest pain, most cases of chest pain aren't due to heart attacks. Thus, the probability that a patient has chest pain given that he has a myocardial infarction (P[B/A]) is very different from the probability that he has a myocardial infarction given that he has chest pain (P[A/B]). The dangers of assuming that P[A/B] = P[B/A] are readily apparent. This is a manifestation of the problems that most individuals have when confronted with statistical data in the form of conditional probabilities.[38]

It's simply a logical fallacy to believe that a conditional probability may be substituted for its inverse without altering the meaning the expression.

(iii) Alternatively, the P-value may be taken for the probability that the results observed were due to chance.[20] Once again, though, this is false. If H_0 is true, the samples are drawn from the same population and, hence, any difference observed must be due to sampling error – that is, the difference observed is due to chance. Put another way, the P-value depends on the assumption that the probability of the data being due to chance is 1. The P-value can't, therefore, be interpreted as the probability of the data being due to chance.[20]

(iv) For those who make the mistake of interpreting the P-value as the probability that H_0 is true, it's a short step to assume that (1 – P-value) is the probability that the alternative hypothesis is true. This

Misunderstandings and Misinterpretations

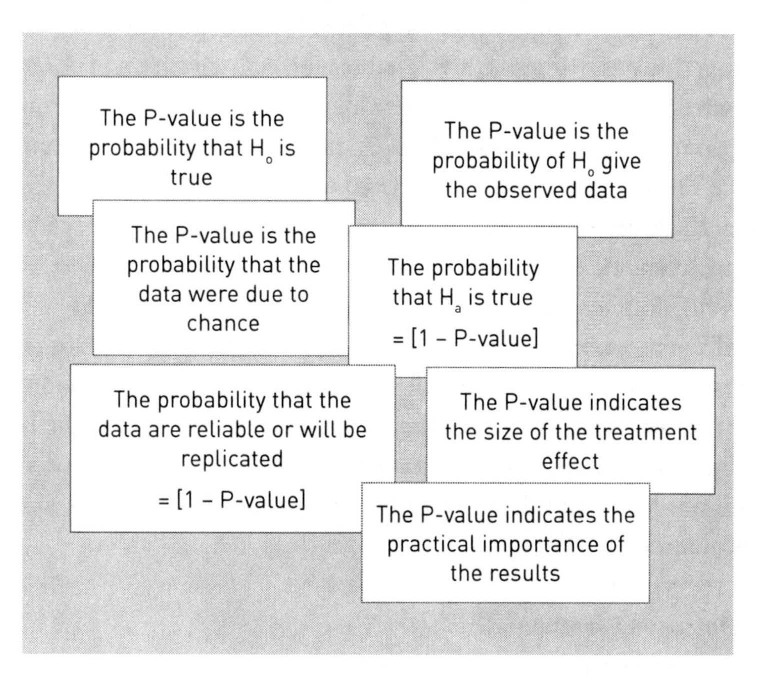

error, it seems, isn't unusual.[24,27,31-33] The argument appears to be that if $P[H_0]$ is known and if it's assumed that H_0 and H_a are mutually exclusive, $P[H_a]$ may be calculated directly. But, the P-value is not $P[H_0]$. Hence the P-value cannot be used to calculate $P[H_a]$.

(v) Others make the mistake of believing that the P-value is somehow related to the replication of data in future trials.[39] Although many have argued that such a view is wrong,[16,20] others believe that a small P-value supports the claim that future studies will show similar results.[33] The source of this error lies in taking (1 – P-value) to be a measure of the reliability of the data and, hence, that the outcome will be replicated in future experiments. But the P-value has nothing to do with reliability or replication. They are different concepts altogether.

(vi) From the point of view of interpreting research data, believing that small P-values indicate large treatment effects is a serious mistake. The size of the P-value isn't directly related to size of the treatment effect.[27] A large study may report a low P-value with only a very small difference in outcome between the groups while a small sample may report a marginal or non-significant P-value in the face of a large treatment effect. The P-value, however, is related to the size of the treatment effect when the sample size and variance are held constant.[33,45] In general, it's wrong to equate the P-value with the size of the treatment effect.

(vii) While statistical significance isn't the same as clinical significance, many people believe that a P-value of <0.05 means that the treatment effect is of practical importance. But a large study may report a very low P-value despite the treatment difference being trivial as shown in the numerous mega-trials published nowadays. Attention has been drawn to this problem for many years [20,33,45] but the mistake continues to be common.

The focus on P-values

Not only is the choice of a cut-off for the P-value at 0.05 entirely arbitrary but adopting it as a convention has had unfortunate consequences.[14] It encourages an unthinking, automatic response to reject or fail to reject H_0. To all intents and purposes, the difference between P=0.045 and P=0.055 is of no importance yet the P-value of 0.05 dictates whether or not the results of a study are statistically significant.[33] On such small margins, the efficacy of treatment may be decided.

The emphasis on P-values draws attention away from the size of the samples studied and the magnitude of the treatment effect observed. Indeed, some have argued that, for any given P-value, the evidence against H_0 is stronger for smaller studies than for larger ones.[42,46-49] As already discussed, large studies with small effects have the same P-values as small studies with large effects, yet large effects are clearly more clinically important than small ones. None of this, though, is reflected in P-values. Whilst it may be argued that the information regarding the size of either the sample or the treatment effect are available in the published study, this ignores the way in which the statistical significance has become the deciding factor. It's now the final word on the interpretation of the results of a study.

The issue of "more extreme" data

As we've seen, the definition of the P-value isn't simply the probability of the data given H_0, but the probability of data at least as extreme as those observed in the trial given H_0. Fisher argued that if a particular result provided evidence against H_0, then it followed that any result more extreme – that is, a result further out into the tail of the distribution given H_0 – would also be evidence against H_0.

This, though, creates a problem. How is the term *more extreme* to be defined? Perhaps surprisingly, the answer to this question includes consideration of the intentions of the investigators.[13,32,44,50]

Berger and Berry gave the example of tossing a coin 17 times and observing 13 heads and four tails, the fourth tail occurring on the final toss.[44] The statistical significance of this outcome depends on what the investigators intended at the start of the study. They may, for example, have simply planned to toss the coin 17 times and test the outcome; in this case, the P-value would be 0.05. On the other hand, they may have decided to toss the coin until they had obtained four heads and four tails; the probability of the endpoint being reached on the 17th toss would be 0.02. The sample is the same and the observed outcome is the same but the P-value is different. This is because the different intentions produce different underlying populations. One comprises all possible outcomes of 17 tosses whilst the other is all of the outcomes that finish with a result that completes four heads and four tails. Clearly, unlike the first population, the second is not limited in size.[33,44]

Since the intentions of investigators vary, what is understood by "more extreme" also varies. Different intentions lead to different sets of possible "more extreme" outcomes which affect the P-values. Thus, the statistical analysis of the results of a trial may produce different conclusions.

But the concept of more extreme outcomes is essential for the frequency approach. If the outcome to be tested is a single point, its probability may be very small no matter where it occurs in the distribution. Consider the example discussed by Lindley.[50] An unbiased coin is tossed ten times in succession and the result observed is TTHTHHHTHT – in other words a sequence amounting to five heads and five tails. The probability of this specific outcome is <0.001, although, of course, we would accept this result as being due to chance. Fisher's solution was to take the data in terms of an area under the distribution curve for values equal to or more extreme than the observed result. This manoeuvre increases the probability of the result because it includes all possible values in that interval. But this introduces the problems related to the intentions of investigators. Furthermore, the tail areas of the distribution curves under H_0 are hypothetical. Hence the P-values depend on data that were not actually observed.[14,44,50]

Currently, the problems associated with the idea of more extreme data are viewed as being an important challenge to frequentist statistics.[50]

Confidence intervals – a genuine alternative to P-values?

Almost from the outset, P-values have been viewed with suspicion by some statisticians. Within twenty years of their appearance, there were calls for alternatives to this method of analysing statistical data, the most common proposal being to supplement or even replace P-values with confidence intervals.[33,51] Over recent decades, more and more medical journals have insisted that confidence intervals be included in research publications. Confidence intervals are believed to have advantages over P-values including, for example, that they present data in such a way that we may appreciate more readily the size of the treatment effect, that they provide an indication of the uncertainty of this estimate, and that they allow for a degree of interpretation.

It would be a mistake, however, to believe that confidence intervals are free from the problems associated with P-values.[13,14] Like P-values, they're derived from frequentist statistics and so share the same underlying weaknesses.[13,33,52-54] For example, they use the 5% cut-off for statistical significance and, thus, include an arbitrary component. They're equally liable to misinterpretation.[14] Contrary to popular belief, the 95% confidence interval doesn't mean that there's a 95% chance that the parameter is located within the interval. Instead, it refers to the frequency with which the statistical test, if repeated many times, would generate bounds capturing the true but unknown parameter. Confidence intervals also require the same assumptions about random sampling and distributions as other frequentist methods and, if these aren't satisfied, the estimates are invalid.[33]

The emphasis on confidence intervals does little to remove the problems inherent in the frequentist approach to statistical analysis.

In defence of the P-value

That there are numerous misunderstandings isn't a matter of debate. But this doesn't necessarily imply that there's something wrong with P-values. There's plenty of evidence that people have difficulty dealing with conditional probabilities and it's only to be expected that they will find P-values troublesome. This has nothing to do with the validity of the concept of the P-value. However, the fact that misunderstandings are so widespread suggests that people's general appreciation of the statistical approach to research is poor and, therefore, unlikely to allow a critical appraisal of what is involved.[20,31] Perhaps this goes some way to explaining the general failure to scrutinise the statistics involved in medical research. However, some commentators have even gone further and argued that the widespread misunderstandings – including amongst statisticians – suggest that there's something fundamentally wrong with the methodology.[27]

Yet, what's interesting about the misunderstandings is that they all veer away from the correct interpretation in the direction of something that appears to have more meaning than the actual P-value. It's often stated that the P-value doesn't give researchers what they really want.[14,29-31,55] They set out, for example, to determine whether a particular drug leads to an improvement in the outcome of patients. They want to know whether the data from the trial support their hypothesis that there's a treatment effect. More precisely, they want to know $P[H_0/d]$ or, better, $P[H_a/d]$. But the P-value delivers the inverse, $P[d/H_0]$. As Nickerson put it,

> "What the null hypothesis test answers is a question that we never ask: What is the probability of getting an outcome as extreme as the one obtained if the null hypothesis is true?" [33]

Strictly speaking, this is correct. But researchers do want to know whether the results obtained in an experiment should be attributed to chance or, instead, taken as support for the presence of a causal relationship. Fisher's approach is perceived as unsatisfactory because it misses out so much that would be expected of an analysis of the data from an experiment. The P-value gives no information about the size of the treatment effect and it allows no inferences about the probability of any hypothesis given the observed data.

In response, researchers convince themselves that significance testing delivers more than is actually the case. They believe, for example, that a small P-value indicates that the probability of H_0 being true is small. Nickerson argues that this is acceptable[33] and is supported by Berger and Sellke.[24] However, these arguments are based on assumptions and we can never be certain that they hold.

As will be argued shortly, it's possible to offer a defence of Fisher's P-value. But, what can't be denied is that its introduction has sown much confusion, that it has led to an over-emphasis on the importance of the results of statistical analysis and that the problems related to the issue of more extreme data seem intractable. Moreover, the P-value is intimately bound up with the even more troublesome notion of the null hypothesis.

The obscurity of the null hypothesis

The null hypothesis is unsettling. From our first acquaintance with it, we're left feeling as though we've missed the point. It seems nothing more than a nuisance and the dissatisfaction never quite leaves us.

> "We psychologists all learned about hypothesis testing during our undergraduate days. Many of us remember thinking at the time that it seemed kind of backward and perverse. No one ever seemed to know exactly what hypothesis testing could tell you that was at all interesting or important. Many budding psychologists... came to believe in a variety of murky and generally incorrect implications of the process... Somewhere along the line, however, we all internalized one lesson that is entirely correct: the more you reject the null hypothesis, the more likely it is that you'll get tenure." [35]

Understanding the concepts related to the null hypothesis is far from easy.[45] For example, it may appear to us that, if we fail to reject H_0, it's reasonable to claim that H_0 is true. We have to learn that this is not the case. We can't speak of the truth of H_0 in such circumstances. When we come face to face with the null hypothesis, we encounter a new language.[56]

Confusions about H_0 are to be found in the earliest textbooks on the subject published in the 1940's [1] and there's little evidence that things have improved with the passage of time.[33] The frequentist approach forces us to live with the null hypothesis and so to put up with the misunderstandings it encourages, the uncomfortable questions it raises and the puzzles it leaves unresolved.

Fisher's use of the null hypothesis

For Fisher, the fundamental problem – and the one which he believed was successfully addressed by frequentist statistics – was to exclude chance as an explanation for the findings of an experiment.[6,10] Discussing a trial which reported that the addition of manure increased the output in a field of one acre by 10% compared with that in another field of the same size left untreated, he enquired:

> "What reason is there to think that, even if no manure had been applied, the acre which actually received it would not still have given the higher yield?" [10]

In other words, given that we have incomplete knowledge of all the factors affecting the yield of crops, how do we know that the result reflects the effect of treatment rather than simply a difference in other factors between the two fields? To answer this, we need a measure of what would be expected if there were no effect from the intervention so that we can compare this with the observed result.

Fisher's solution, as we have seen, is the significance test which depends on H_0. We compare the observed data with the distribution of outcomes that would occur if the experiment were repeated many times and there were no difference between the groups. This is the distribution of differences given the truth of H_0.

When, as is often the case, this method is criticised on the grounds that it fails to provide what researchers actually want, it seems that this is based on a misunderstanding. It's as if the only thing that matters about an experiment is the statistical analysis. But this isn't so.

A trial is designed and performed with the intention of detecting a difference in outcome between different groups. If, as is believed, the conditions for internal validity are satisfied up to the point of statistical significance, then a great deal has been achieved already. We know, for example, that the groups are matched in terms of all other relevant factors for the outcome apart from the treatment given; and we know that the assessment of the outcome is not subject to bias. Thus, before the statistical analysis, we may say that any observed difference between the groups is the result of treatment provided that it's not due to chance. This is where the statisticians have their role. They are to answer the straightforward question: is the result due to chance? And it follows that the P-value is precisely what is required in this situation.

Fisher's solution must be seen as an integral part of the process by which we identify causal relationships and is to be used in conjunction with the other criteria for internal validity. But, in constructing his tests of significance, he was obliged to introduce the null hypothesis with its unwelcome baggage.

A misunderstanding: if P>0.05, then Ho is true

Just as in the case of P-values, there are misunderstandings about the null hypothesis. A frequent mistake is to believe that if the null hypothesis isn't rejected, then it's true.[33]

The error may expressed as follows: if the statistical analysis of an observed difference shows that $P>0.05$, then H_0 isn't rejected; if H_0 isn't rejected, then H_0 is true. But here, we should remember that the nature of the cut-off level for statistical significance is arbitrary; it's merely a convention. Drawing such a boundary produces unacceptable consequences. For instance, $P = 0.045$ leads to rejection of H_0 while $P = 0.055$ doesn't, despite there being only a trivial difference between the two measures. If this is accepted, then it follows that a P-value of 0.055 leading to the failure to reject H_0 could hardly be said to provide strong evidence in favour of H_0, let alone justify claims to the truth of H_0. The basic point is that there's no symmetry around the cut off point such that H_0 is false on one side and true on the other. By convention, a P-value just below 0.05 is sufficient to reject H_0 but the same convention entails nothing about the acceptance of H_0 if we find the P-value is >0.05.

There's another argument against this view and this relates to the power of a study. A small trial may show a difference in outcome between the groups although this difference fails to achieve statistical significance because the number of participants is too low. While the decision not to reject H_0 is correct, it would be wrong to infer from this that H_0 is true.[33,56]

Of course, other flaws with internal validity – for example, unequal distribution of relevant factors – may reduce the size of the observed difference and yield a higher P-value than would otherwise have been the case, thus leading to a failure to reject H_0 even when it is false. This, though, isn't a problem of frequentist statistics.[33,56]

In any case, we can't logically infer the truth of H_0 from the P-value. If we recall that the P-value is $P[d/H_0]$, we see that it can't be grounds for inferring that H_0 is true. Any such inference would involve exchanging $P[d/H_0]$ for $P[H_0/d]$ which can't be achieved by frequentist methods.

Fisher was clear that we shouldn't use the expression "accepting the null hypothesis". We're only entitled to speak of rejecting or not rejecting H_0. In this regard, he was surely correct. There are no grounds for asserting that a failure to reject H_0 entails that it is true.

Can we ever say that Ho is true?

Both significance tests and hypothesis tests assume the truth of the null hypothesis. But can we ever say that H_0 is true? Many writers have argued that such a claim is false.[16,29,37,39,55,57-59] They point out that, in any experiment, it's very unlikely that there'll be no difference – no matter how small – between the groups and even very small differences can be shown to be statistically significant provided that the sample size is large enough. This is disturbing because it threatens the results of experiments that fail to reject H_0. By increasing the size of the sample, the decision regarding H_0 would be reversed. H_0 is, therefore, never true. But, if this is the case, where does it leave the P-value which is conditional on the truth of H_0?

Many others disagree and believe that it's wrong to say that H_0 is never true.[33] They draw attention to the fact that samples taken from the same population will be likely to show small differences. Hence, the presence of a difference can't be said to imply that the samples were taken from different populations.[33,60] This is relevant because H_0, by definition, entails that the samples are drawn from the same population. We only speak of rejecting H_0 when the difference between samples reaches a specified level of statistical significance. Thus, any observed difference is compatible with either the samples coming from the same population or from different populations and the conclusion we reach is determined by statistical analysis. If the difference fails to reach a specified level of significance, we don't infer anything other than that we're not in a position to reject H_0. In this situation, we can't comment on the truth or falsity of H_0.

Those who believe that H_0 is never true argue that if a difference is found that fails to reach statistical significance, then simply by increasing the sample size in a further experiment we'll be able to show a low P-value and, hence, reject H_0. But a non-significant difference can't be taken as providing support for the belief that H_0 is false. It just leaves us in limbo. We certainly can't assume that a larger study will convert a non-significant difference into a significant one – for all we know, the new data may even show that the direction of the difference is reversed.

Null hypothesis testing – the ideal situation

As we saw earlier, misunderstandings and confusions are no strangers to frequentist statistics. But, just as with the P-value, they don't justify abandoning the use of H_0. Researchers continue to compare data with the distribution of differences under H_0 and the scientific community, in general, accepts the methodology.

Our initial encounter with significance testing focuses on the P-value. It takes time to become accustomed to, and feel comfortable with, this concept. After wrestling with the P-value, the last thing we want to do is to suffer the torment of delving more deeply into the null hypothesis. Perhaps we just settle for accepting the idea of comparing the data with the distribution of differences under H_0 in order to determine whether the results of an experiment are due to chance. After all, it's simply like finding a particular shade of red using a colour chart, isn't it? The analogy, however, only works so far. We know what it is to get hold of a colour chart but obtaining the distribution of differences under H_0 isn't so straightforward.

When we think about null hypothesis testing, we may have in mind the example of a game of chance. Imagine that someone claimed that he was able to influence the outcome of a toss of a coin so that he could increase the proportion of heads. To try to prove to him that his claim is false, we design an experiment in which he selects a coin at random from a large urn – to exclude the possibility of biased coins – and tosses it, repeating the selection and the toss 1000 times. The outcome is 510 heads and 490 tails, giving a proportion of heads of 0.51. Does this result support his claim? To decide this, we compare the result with the distribution of outcomes expected if H_0 is true. With an unbiased coin, the probability of heads is 0.5 and from this, together with the number of tosses, we can calculate the variance using the binomial method. Thus, the probability distribution of possible outcomes under H_0 is known a priori and is independent of the results of the experiment. The comparison of the observed data with the distribution of outcomes under H_0 is easy. We simply read off the probability of a result at least as large as that observed.

This is the ideal scenario for thinking about null hypothesis testing. Everything is cut and dried. The frequency distribution of the statistic given that H_0 is true is known a priori. And, throughout, there's a consistent position with respect to H_0. We believe in the truth of H_0 at the start, during the statistical analysis and at the end of the experiment – even if the P-value is very small. It would take much more than a single experiment to overturn our beliefs about the outcome of coin-tossing. But this is a special case.

When null hypothesis testing is brought into question

The situation is altogether different in RCTs. If we go to the trouble and expense of designing and carrying out a large-scale trial, we do so because we have reason to believe that a difference will be found. We may have theoretical grounds for believing this or, alternatively, we may be aware of experimental evidence from other studies using other similar drugs or the same drug in similar clinical settings. We only have to read the protocol of any RCT to learn about the grounds for expecting a treatment benefit. Thus, the starting position is the belief that there will be a treatment effect – we believe H_0 is false.

What is the distribution of differences under Ho?

The way in which significance testing is described suggests that finding the distribution of differences under H_0 is little more than a formality. The mean of the differences is, by definition, zero. But, unlike the coin experiment, we can't determine the variance of the differences a priori and, instead, we have to use the data collected during the trial. The variance of the difference is obtained by combining the variance of the data in the active treatment group and that in the placebo group.

Consider the two possible outcomes:

(a) The observed difference in outcome is not statistically significant. In this case, H_0 isn't rejected and the two samples are said to have been drawn from the same population. Apart from sampling error, there's no reason to believe that the variance of the data in the active treatment group will be different from that in the placebo group. Under these conditions, the combination of the two variances is taken to be an estimate of the variance of the differences under H_0. Here, the process of significance testing appears to be satisfactory. In many respects, it resembles the coin experiment.

(b) The observed difference in outcome is found to be statistically significant and H_0 is rejected. The samples, therefore, have been drawn from different populations. In the circumstances, we can't assume that the variance of the data in the two groups will be the same and, hence, pooling the data may not provide a reliable estimate of the variance of the difference under H_0.

If H_0 is rejected, the resemblance to the coin experiment is lost. Before the trial, H_0 is believed to be false; during the statistical analysis, this belief is suspended and H_0 is assumed to be true; at the end, H_0 is rejected. As a consequence, the attitude to the number of populations present also changes: at first, there are two; then we assume there's one; and finally we accept that there are two populations.

Here, we have a problem. The aim of the analysis is to determine whether the result obtained in the RCT was due to a treatment effect or occurred by chance. To achieve this, we compare the difference observed with the distribution of differences if there were no treatment effect – in other words, if H_0 were true. But the data used to construct this distribution were derived from two populations, not one. How, then, can we say that we compared the difference in outcome with the distribution under H_0? Of course, we fall back on the observation that the variance of the two samples is similar and the belief that this doesn't affect the analysis. But this doesn't detract from the uneasiness created by a situation in which, at the same time, we accept both that the observed difference was, and that it was not, compared with the distribution of differences under H_0. This has implications, too, for the meaning of the P-value which depends on the truth of H_0 and, thus, on the presence of a single population.

The null hypothesis is central to frequentist statistics. But it's an obscure, slippery concept that produces muddle and confusion.

The Fisher-Neyman-Pearson hybrid

One of the more unsatisfactory developments over the past 50 years has been the merger of Fisher's significance tests with the Neyman-Pearson hypothesis test.[13,61,62] Nowadays, the distinction between the two procedures is lost. We commonly see publications of medical research which include elements of each approach.

Fisher, as well as Neyman and Pearson, were opposed to any fusion because of the fundamental differences between the two methods. Their advice, however, has been ignored and significance testing is routinely mixed with hypothesis tests. According to Goodman,[13] this hybrid version has its origins in the need to address the weakness of the hypothesis test, namely, that it doesn't provide a measure of the strength of evidence for or against the hypothesis. By incorporating the P-value into trials designed along the lines of the hypothesis test, the conclusions are believed to support the presence of a causal relationship between treatment and outcome. But the P-value was never intended to be part of the hypothesis test.[13,63]

The mixing together of two fundamentally different approaches to statistical analysis has inevitably led to unwanted consequences.[13,61,62] For example, it produces confusion between the P-value and the Type I error rate, alpha. Both relate to the tail areas of probability distribution curves and both are frequently associated with a value of 0.05. But they are very different. Alpha is selected before the trial begins and refers to the long-run probability of committing a Type I error. The P-value, on the other hand, depends on the data collected during the trial and represents the strength of evidence against H_0. The trouble arises when these distinctions become blurred.

Goodman refers to the "P-value fallacy" by which he means the belief that an event can be viewed both from the long-run and the short-run perspectives at the same time. This, he argues forcibly, isn't possible.[13] The confusions and inconsistencies resulting from the P-value fallacy are the source of many of the statistical problems associated with frequentist methods. This applies, in particular, to the case of multiple comparisons where there are well-recognised difficulties in calculating the correct P-values. For instance, in subgroup analysis, there's no straightforward answer to the question of whether the results of each comparison are to be considered individually and treated as separate statistical problems or to be taken collectively and the subsequent P-values corrected for multiple comparisons.[13,63]

The hybrid version shows how easy it is for mistakes to occur in the development of statistical methods and, equally, how easy it is for flawed methods to become widely accepted. Not everyone is fooled, of course. The flaws are well recognised by academic statisticians but, as will be familiar by now, concerns about statistical theory seldom surface in non-specialist textbooks or journals.

Assumptions inherent in statistical tests

As discussed at the beginning of this chapter, statistics concerns inferences about populations or, more specifically, about population parameters. In most circumstances, we have no knowledge of the true values of these parameters. Instead, we use the data from experiments to make estimates of the value of the parameters in order to permit further inference.

Statistical tests involve assumptions. For example, when comparing the means of two samples, it's assumed that the samples are selected randomly, that the population from which they are drawn is normally distributed and that they have approximately the same variance. But as to the true distribution of the population – its mean and standard deviation – we know nothing. As already mentioned, there are procedures that may be used to determine whether or not these assumptions have been met. It's seldom clear, however, that the assumptions have been tested. Nickerson, for example, believes that such procedures are usually omitted.[33]

The failure to ensure that the assumptions underlying statistical tests are satisfied is of particular relevance to observational studies. In this situation, random sampling and the random allocation of treatment are missing. Somehow, though, this is overlooked and statistical analysis is performed as if the data were obtained from a standard randomised controlled trial.[64] But if the assumptions aren't satisfied, we can have little confidence in the outcome of the statistical analysis[64] and, hence, in the validity of epidemiological studies. But there's another consequence. Once again, we encounter a situation in which statistical analysis involving frequentist methods is flawed. At the very least, this raises doubts about other decisions made by medical researchers and statisticians.

Bias in frequentist statistics

It's not uncommon to hear it said that that the frequentist method is biased in favour of the rejection of H_0.[29,50,65-69]

Those who believe that H_0 is always false argue that a statistically significant difference will be found provided that the size of the study is increased sufficiently. A point null hypothesis – that is, one specifying a particular value for the outcome, usually zero – will nearly always be false because of the nature of the data in the biological sciences as well as in fields such as psychology and sociology.[29] Thus, by chance, a difference will be observed in the direction of H_a in at least 50% of studies.[65]

But there is an asymmetry with respect to H_0 and H_a. We've already noted how the failure to reject H_0 doesn't permit any statement to be made about the truth of H_0. Thus, frequentist methods only allow for one definite conclusion – the rejection of H_0.[29] Given that researchers generally believe the truth of H_a and, hence, the falsity of H_0, a failure to reject H_0 is usually attributed to other flaws in internal validity and this allows them to avoid confronting the possibility that H_0 is true.[29]

These arguments suggesting bias in the statistical analysis are debatable. But there's another which is more convincing and deserves serious attention.[69] Goodman describes how frequentist methods overestimate the statistical significance of the difference detected in an experiment. He compares the strength of evidence according to Bayesian analysis with that of P-values. For example, a P-value of 0.05 gives an equivalent figure of 0.15 with the Bayes factor. Thus the significance level is exaggerated by conventional statistical techniques and, consequently, the strength of evidence against H_0 is nowhere near as great as we are led to believe by the P-value. It should be pointed out, however, that the two methods produce more similar results as the P-values become very small.

As will be discussed later in this chapter, Bayesian methods tend to produce more conservative estimates of the strength of evidence because they incorporate prior knowledge. However, Goodman's argument doesn't involve the use of other evidence and so the discrepancy between the strength of evidence according to the P-value and that derived from Bayesian analysis can't be attributed to the effect of priors.

Whether or not we agree with Goodman depends on our willingness to accept Bayesian analysis. But, at the very least, it casts doubt on the reliability of P-values as a measure of the strength of evidence against H_0.

Frequentist theories and objectivity

We've already seen how Fisher accepted an element of subjectivity into scientific research. This prompted Neyman and Pearson to develop hypothesis testing in an attempt to eradicate any hint of interpretation in the analysis of experimental data. Unfortunately, this led to the widespread acceptance of a methodology devoid of any flexibility. The process is automatic and the 0.05 level dictates the response.

Many scientists assert the objectivity of their subject. Frequently, however, this isn't the case in practice. In a provocative paper, Matthews points to many instances of overt subjectivity in different scientific disciplines.[14] It appears that scientists want it both ways. This may be seen in the often inconsistent responses of researchers to essentially the same strength of evidence. For example, while a study of passive smoking and lung cancer was interpreted as supporting a causal link, a report of the association between electric power lines and leukaemia was dismissed as showing no causal relationship. In each case, the evidence was the same: the size of the odds ratio was similar and neither of the results was statistically significant. Yet the similarities failed to prevent the researchers from reporting the data in line with both their preconceived ideas and the orthodox views of the research community.[14]

Goodman, too, has drawn attention to the subjective interpretation of frequentist statistics.[13] When it suits researchers, they'll interpret the P-value rigidly but, at other times, they'll adopt a more flexible approach. An expected or favourable result, with unimpressive statistical significance, is greeted with enthusiasm while an unexpected or unfavourable result – even if it's statistically significant – is deemed to be a fluke and rejected.[13]

Despite all the talk of objectivity in science, it seems that – in the context of statistical studies, at least – this only matters when it's convenient.

Failure to take background knowledge into account

The frequentist method is often criticised on the grounds that it provides no formal process by which pre-existing knowledge may influence the interpretation of the results. Indeed, background knowledge plays little part in the inferences drawn from the data.[13] This particular criticism, however, is usually levelled by Bayesians who, given the central role which they assign to prior probabilities, understandably wish to emphasize what they see as an advantage to their approach.

Nonetheless, the subject matter of medical research based on statistics is such that the interpretation of the results of any one study would appear to benefit from taking into account what is already known. Fisher, for example, believed that the data should not be judged in isolation. Neyman and Pearson, on the other hand, adopted a method that focused entirely on accepting the verdict of the hypothesis testing procedure. The consequence of frequentist theories is that the statistical aspect takes precedence over other considerations.[13]

Reasons for acceptance of frequentist theories

Frequentist theories arrived on the scene at just the right moment. The first half of the 20th century was characterised by the search for objectivity in science [13,70] as may be seen, for example, in the works of Rudolf Carnap and Karl Popper. There was a belief that subjectivity could be eradicated, that interpretation was a relic of the past, and that the entire process could be governed by a rigid methodology with decisions no longer dependent on researchers.[70] It was in this climate that statistics – and, more particularly, the frequentist school – was keenly embraced.

Gigerenzer described the way in which psychology was rapidly taken over by statistics.[1] By the mid-1950s, 80% of published papers used frequentist statistics and this proportion has increased to almost 100% in recent times. Medicine, too, found statistics irresistible. Frequentists offered cures for all of the ills affecting medical research. Advocates of the new approach encouraged ever larger studies to seek out smaller effects that made statistics indispensable to epidemiologists and clinical researchers alike. The frequentist approach captured the market in medical research early on. By the 1960's, it had a monopoly, with editors of journals rejecting any papers submitted without the mandatory P-value.[28,32,33] In undergraduate and postgraduate medical education, too, the frequentist theory has been in control from the start.[28,32]

The frequentist school went from strength to strength. It was seen to provide a degree of objectivity previously unheard of in medical research. The tables of numerical values, the mathematical symbols and the obscure formulae all contributed to giving epidemiological studies and RCTs an air of respectability.[20,28,33] As in the social sciences, so too in medicine, the merest hint of statistical analysis using P-values or confidence intervals was enough to stifle all argument. A study yielding results that were statistically significant wasn't to be questioned. The effect had been demonstrated and that was the end of the matter.

Medical research had become a true scientific discipline – at least, that's what was believed.

Marks offers a different interpretation of the success of frequentist methods.[70] He argues that the eagerness to accept statistics was a reaction to the growing mistrust of doctors, researchers and pharmaceutical companies that emerged during the first half of the 20th century.[70]

But there's another reason for the success of frequentist statistics. Goodman and others have drawn attention to the way in which an objective, investigator-independent approach to medical research is appealing to those seeking reform in health care systems.[13,70,71] For the government, it's obviously an advantage to have available an approach to research that can be controlled by those outside of the medical profession and one which produces information that isn't open to debate. Managers want clear-cut, simple, easily intelligible answers, free from the interpretation that for so long has been the prerogative of the medical profession. Decisions can then be made without the interference of doctors. They can be based on guidelines and followed by nurses, health care assistants or anyone else who harbours ideas of practicing medicine without confronting the obstacles of medical school and a protracted period of post-graduate education. And there is, in the eyes of politicians and NHS managers, a desirable side-effect of the process – the weakening of the role of the medical profession.

Frequentist statistics with its promotion of objectivity is fundamental to many of the health service reforms. It supplies the ammunition for those who want to argue that epidemiological studies and RCTs provide knowledge and that the results should simply be followed without question.

The verdict on frequentist statistics

Frequentist statisticians have skilfully created the illusion that all is well with their activities. Their textbooks consistently avoid any mention of internal disputes [1,45] and the apparent consensus has been achieved by air-brushing away any dissent.[1,35,45] When faced with external challenges, they point to the widespread adoption of their methods and claim that this supports their case – surely it's inconceivable that the millions of researchers and academics who use tests of significance and hypothesis tests could all be wrong? Yet, as we've seen, misunderstandings and confusions about the basic components of frequentist statistics are endemic. If, as studies suggest, this applies to those involved in research, then they're hardly in a position to appraise critically the fundamental features of the method and, consequently, their support is of little value. The general acceptance of these methods isn't necessarily evidence of their validity. Thus, the advocates of frequentist statistics are more exposed than might, at first sight, appear. To an impartial observer, the weight of criticism of frequentist statistics is telling.

The history of frequentist statistics is characterised by the emergence of flaws in the methods that have been accepted unquestioningly into routine practice for many years. This is a recurring theme. Multiple comparisons have been performed for decades without the appropriate statistical corrections and this has led to numerous false-positive and false-negative findings. The hybrid version involving both tests of significance and hypothesis testing appears regularly in the journals despite recognition of the problems resulting from the mixing together of two fundamentally different approaches. And researchers persist in using statistical methods in epidemiological studies that are suitable only for randomised controlled trials. How many more errors in frequentist statistics are awaiting discovery?

The problems associated with the use of more extreme data, the uncertainties surrounding the distribution of differences under the null hypothesis, the failure to satisfy the assumptions for statistical tests, the bias in favour of rejection of H_0 and the exaggerated level of statistical significance raise serious doubts about the inferences derived from frequentist methods. Individually, these flaws are troublesome; collectively, they are crippling to frequentist statistics.

Criticism of Frequentist Statistics

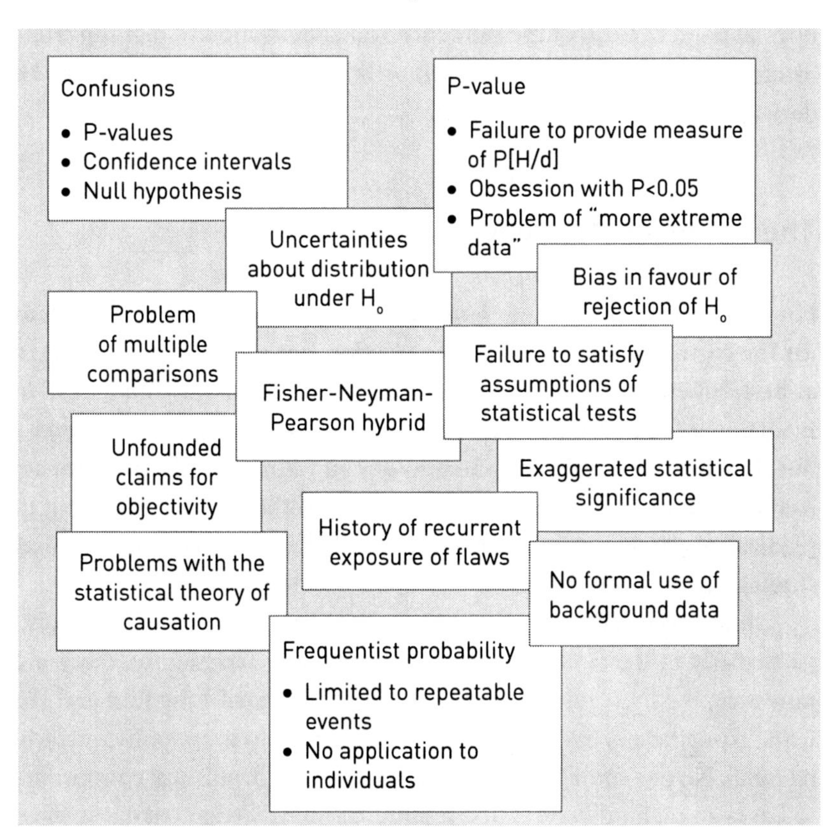

But even if we were able to dismiss these concerns, there remain questions about the very foundations of tests of significance and hypothesis tests. As noted earlier, the frequentist theory of probability may be criticised on the grounds that it fails to provide a broad theory of probability and that its inferences don't apply to individuals. And, at a deeper level, the inferences drawn from experimental data rely on the statistical approach to causation which is far from being unproblematic.

The conventional approach to statistics in research is under threat on so many fronts that it's to be wondered how it can survive. That it does so is a reflection of the influence and effectiveness of its supporters in creating a façade of success rather than any genuine benefit to be derived from the methodology.

The Bayesian Approach

For many years, Bayesian methods have been advocated as a replacement for the conventional approach to statistics. But the response has been, at best, lukewarm. Bayesians have had an influence on some areas of medicine – for example, in assessing the accuracy of diagnostic tests – but elsewhere, especially in epidemiology and clinical trials, their impact has been all but non-existent.[3,72] A review of the literature relating to medical research between 1990 and 1998 identified very few clinical studies which involved the use of Bayesian statistics.[3]

More recently, though, there has been increasing interest, particularly in the field of health economics, and Bayesian methods are now accepted by regulatory authorities in the United Kingdom and the USA.[5] Nonetheless, frequentist statistics continue to monopolise medical research. No one should be surprised. To convert the medical community to Bayesian methods would first require an acknowledgment of the flaws of the frequentist approach. This isn't going to happen in the near future. There's too much at stake – too many individuals and institutions with vested interests in the preservation of the status quo. But there's another obstacle. Researchers would have to undergo a fundamental change in the way they approach probability and statistics.

Bayesian probability

From the Bayesian perspective, probability is a measure of the strength of an individual's belief in the occurrence of an uncertain event.[2] Thus, it's subjective. It depends on the presence of a human mind and varies among different people and in the same people at different times.

The Bayesian approach has important consequences. It makes probability statements and statistical analysis applicable to a much wider range of events than in the case of the frequentist approach which is confined to repeatable events. And it also means that the interpretation of statistical tests is different. Gone is the obsession with speaking of the results in relation to the long-run relative frequency. Instead, the outcome of statistical analysis becomes more straightforward and in line with common sense. But there's another important feature of Bayesian probability. It provides a means by which background knowledge may be formally incorporated into the inferences drawn from the data of an experiment or clinical trial. Indeed, Bayesians consider that the notion of drawing conclusions without taking into consideration pre-existing knowledge is simply wrong. Accordingly, they insist that no result is to be considered in isolation and that previous knowledge must be used in the judgment of causation.[3-5]

The Bayesian method

Given that Bayesian probability is the strength of an individual's belief, it's easy to see how probability will vary according to the data available. But how are pre-existing data to be formally incorporated into inferences drawn from the results of a study? By how much is the strength of a belief to be altered by new data?

The answer was given by Thomas Bayes in the *Essay Towards Solving a Problem in the Doctrine of Chances*,[73] published posthumously in 1764. If we consider two events, A and B, that are not independent, the probability of their occurrence together is determined by the general multiplication rule:

$$P[A \text{ and } B] = P[A].P[B/A]$$

In other words, the probability of the occurrence of both events equals the probability that event A occurs multiplied by the probability that event B occurs given that A occurs. Since P[A and B] = P[B and A],

$$P[A].P[B/A] = P[B].P[A/B]$$

And, from this, we may derive Bayes' theorem.

$$P[B/A] = \frac{P[B].P[A/B]}{P[A]}$$

If we substitute H (the hypothesis) and d (the data observed in the experiment or clinical trial) for B and A, respectively, then Bayes' theorem may be expressed as:

$$P[H/d] = \frac{P[H].P[d/H]}{P[d]}$$

To understand how new data are used to update the probability of a hypothesis, consider further the components of this equation.

(a) P[H]

This is the probability of the hypothesis being true before the trial. It's based on what is known about the subject in advance. In Bayesian statistics, probability is expressed in terms of distribution curves. The outcome of interest is a parameter (θ) – for example, the difference in means or proportions of the outcome between the treatment groups. Pre-existing knowledge allows the construction of a curve showing the expected probabilities for a range of values of θ. This curve is the prior distribution of probabilities.

For instance, before the trial, the information available may suggest that the most likely difference in outcome between the active treatment and the placebo groups is 25%. Accordingly, this and similar results will be given a high probability, whereas values for θ of much less or much greater than 25% will be given low probabilities. The probabilities for each possible value of θ are presented in the form of a distribution curve.

(b) P[d/H]

In the same way, Bayesian statistics presents the probability of observing the data given the hypothesis in terms of a probability distribution. This describes the strength of the evidence from the study data for various values of the parameter.

P[d/H] is known as the likelihood function. This depends exclusively on the observations made during the study. In contrast to the frequentist approach which uses hypothetical data points, the Bayesian likelihood function is calculated only from the observed data.

(c) P[d]

This is the probability of observing the data given all hypotheses. Since the area under the probability distribution curves is adjusted to equal one, P[d] cancels out of the equation.

(d) P[H/d]

The aim of Bayesian analysis is to calculate the probability of the hypothesis, given both the pre-existing data and the data from the trial. This is known as the posterior probability. Once again, it is presented in terms of a probability distribution. The posterior probability distribution is obtained by multiplying the prior probability by the likelihood function for each value of θ.

Prior probabilities

There's no denying that the use of priors is controversial. For the advocates of Bayesian statistics, the inclusion of the prior probability is a crucial strength of their method and a manifest advantage over the frequentist alternative.[3,5] It allows pre-existing knowledge to be taken into account when drawing conclusions about causal relationships from experimental data. But to the frequentists, it's the Achilles heel of the Bayesian challenge because it introduces an unacceptable degree of subjectivity into the process of statistical inference. Different people select different priors even when they have access to the same information.[3]

The source of priors

In principle, prior probability distributions may be based upon any relevant information available before the trial.[14,72] However, Bayesians emphasize that only reliable evidence should be used.[3,5] In medical research, it's rare for there to be no background information. Before any large-scale study, data will be available from animal experiments, pharmacological research in volunteers and pilot studies in patients. In many cases, other trials using the same drug – or one from the same family of drugs – will have been performed in similar diseases.

Priors, though, don't come pre-packaged and have to be constructed. Data from large RCTs or meta-analyses are considered valuable but these may not be available. Moreover, previous trials may have yielded inconsistent results and there may be ongoing disputes about their interpretation. Alternatively, experts may be recruited. Here, though, new problems arise. Elicitation – that is, the process of obtaining information leading to the formation of priors – is unreliable. Experts don't appear to be particularly adept at presenting their conclusions in terms of probability distributions.[5,74]

It's generally agreed that there's no such thing as *the* correct prior probability distribution. Instead, there's a spectrum of priors reflecting a range of views.[74]

The effects of priors

As discussed above, the posterior distribution depends on the prior and the likelihood function. If there's strong evidence before the trial to expect a particular value for the parameter, then the prior distribution curve will contain a sharp peak reflecting the high probability of that value of θ whilst the remaining values will have much lower probabilities. In this situation, the prior will have a powerful effect and move the likelihood curve in its direction. On the other hand, if the data from the trial are strong, the likelihood function will contain a sharp peak indicating a high probability for that value of θ and will move the prior distribution curve in its direction.

Classifications of the different types of priors vary.[5,74] Non-informative or reference priors are selected when there is very limited evidence before the trial and have a flat probability distribution. This means that the prior has little effect on the likelihood and, consequently, the posterior distribution is very close to that of the likelihood function. Enthusiastic priors express a belief in the alternative hypothesis while sceptical priors favour the null hypothesis. The latter are particularly useful in multiple subgroup analysis which, when performed according to frequentist principles, often leads to incorrect conclusions. Sceptical priors demand stronger evidence of an effect and reduce false-positives.

In defence of priors

Bayesians are forthright in their defence of priors.[3,5] When faced with the charge of subjectivity, they present evidence to show that the objectivity purported to be present in the frequentist approach is merely apparent. Whilst this is undoubtedly a challenge to the frequentist approach, the Bayesian *ad hominem* argument does nothing to support their own case for the use of priors.

A better defence is that subjectivity is an integral component of all human activities and, as such, is part and parcel of scientific research. Rather than shying away from it, Bayesians embrace subjectivity and this, of course, is entirely consistent with their view of probability.

In response to disputes about the selection of particular priors, Bayesians propose using a range of different prior distributions. If there's little difference in posterior probabilities over the range, then this approach would appear to have some benefit. On the other hand, if the posterior probabilities differ substantially, then we have to decide which priors to accept. In this case, using a range is hardly an answer to the dispute about the choice of priors in the first place.

Ultimately, Bayesians appear to be able to shrug their shoulders at any criticism of priors because they believe that, as more and more data accumulate, any differences in opinion – expressed formally by prior distributions – will disappear and a consensus will be reached among researchers. In other words, they believe they have a cast iron guarantee of being right in the end.

Bayesian thinking and common sense

Bayesian statistics are claimed to be more in line with common sense than the frequentist alternative. For example, this type of reasoning is said to be natural in decision making in medicine.[75] Gigerenzer, however, argues the opposite case. He provides abundant evidence that educated individuals have difficulty in understanding conditional probabilities.[38] Nevertheless, when dealing with statistics, the concepts involved in the Bayesian approach are closer to common sense than those of the frequentists.

We've seen how Fisher's significance test involved the use of the P-value which was defined as $P[data/H_0]$. But it's often asserted that what the researcher is really interested in is $P[H_0/data]$ or $P[H_a/data]$.[3,14] The Bayesian approach satisfies this requirement by turning the frequentist probabilities upside down and giving researchers a measure more relevant to their purposes.

When it comes to interval estimation, Bayesians again produce something more sensible. Gone is the obscurity associated with frequentist confidence intervals and, in their place, is the simplicity of credible intervals. The definition is exactly what would be expected, namely, that there's a 95% chance that the parameter of interest falls within the 95% credible interval.

Common sense would also dictate that inferences are based solely on data actually observed in the course of the clinical trial. With the frequentist approach, however, this isn't the case. The P-value is the probability of data, the same as or more extreme than those observed in the trial given the truth of the null hypothesis. Thus, the conclusions of research are based, in part, on outcomes that have not been observed. Imaginary data play no part in Bayesian statistics in which the analysis is based only on outcomes that have been observed during the course of the trial.

Advantages of Bayesian statistics

Comprehensive accounts of the advantages of Bayesian statistics over the frequentist approach have been published over recent years.[5,74] Many of the advantages have already been covered in the present chapter and only a brief discussion is required in this section.

Not only are Bayesian methods capable of dealing with questions of probability related to non-repeatable events, but they're not dependent upon randomisation and so have a much wider application than frequentist statistics. Priors offer a way in which pre-existing knowledge may be formally incorporated into drawing inferences from the data, as well as protecting against extreme conclusions. Furthermore, the concepts used in Bayesian statistics are believed to be more in line with common sense.

In recent times, conventional statistics has been dogged by the problem of multiple comparisons. Frequentist statistics offers no clear guidance as to the best method for tackling this issue whereas Bayesians have a ready solution.[3,13,69,74]

More generally, frequentist analysis is believed to produce exaggerated measures of statistical significance when compared with the Bayesian approach. In particular, sceptical priors reduce the statistical significance compared with that reported by frequentist statistics.[14,69]

Advantages of Bayesian Statistics

A general approach to probability
- Not restricted to repeatable events
- Not dependent on randomisation

Priors
- Use of pre-existing knowledge in inference
- Transparency of background data
- Protects against far-fetched conclusions

Common sense
- Terms are straightforward and better understood
- Only uses observed data
- Results presented as P[H/d] rather than P[d/H]

Resolution of problems with conventional statistics
- Solution to multiple comparisons
- Avoids inflated P-values of frequentist methods

Broad application to medical research

Bayesian statistics is claimed to have broad application to medical research. It is, for example, being used increasingly in health economics[5] and decision-making, it's suitable for the statistical analysis of clinical trials and recent advances have enabled it to be applied to epidemiological studies.[74]

Disadvantages of Bayesian statistics

In the face of the many problems with the frequentist approach, it's tempting to accept the arguments of the more enthusiastic advocates of

Bayesian statistics. Criticisms, however, aren't difficult to find [76,77] and some of these are openly acknowledged by Bayesians themselves.[74]

Problems related to prior probabilities

As expected, many of the criticisms of Bayesian statistics focus on the use of priors.

(a) The construction of prior probability distributions is far from straightforward. Difficulties in elicitation of priors from experts are recognised and there's no guarantee that the distributions accurately reflect their views.

(b) Experts are not impartial. They have a point of view, a stance for or against a particular treatment, and this may easily introduce bias into their selection of a particular prior distribution.[74] In this context, it's important to remember that many individuals who would be considered by the medical community to be experts in their field receive payment from pharmaceutical companies. The choice of a particular expert clearly provides an opportunity for those involved in setting up the trial to affect the outcome.[74] For example, it's unlikely that the pharmaceutical industry would select experts offering unfavourable priors. Were Bayesian statistics to become widely used in medical research, the selection of experts would become a major source of dispute.

(c) Priors rest on the notion that previous studies provide reliable data on which the prior distribution may be based. But this isn't the case. We've already discussed the problems that threaten the conclusions of clinical trials. Moreover, the data are often inconsistent. And, of course, they're based on the frequentist approach to statistics which, in the eyes of Bayesians, is flawed. How, then, is it possible to have confidence in priors derived from such insecure sources?

(d) The argument in favour of the use of a range of priors may, in theory, be reasonable but its practical consequences are problematic for Bayesian statistics. If a prior is accepted for inclusion into the study, it must have some validity. But, since this applies to all priors selected, it follows that we may simply choose the posterior that is in our interest and support the decision on the grounds of the prior that produced it. Different camps with different views on the matter will each be able to argue their own position based on interpretations of previous data.

Problems with Bayesian Statistics

Priors

- Difficulties constructing distributions
- Questionable impartiality of experts
- Dispute about reliability of previous studies
- Using a range of priors leaves open a choice of posterior distributions

Subjectivity

Computational problems

Problems understanding conditional probability

Limited experience in medical research

Different schools within Bayesian statistics

Probability theory of causation

Other problems related to Bayesian statistics

Much has been made of subjectivity. Opponents have used it endlessly to torment Bayesians, particularly in relation to the use of priors. In return, Bayesians have attacked the notion of objectivity in frequentist statistics and science in general. In practice, both approaches are subjective. But this isn't so obvious in the case of the frequentist approach. Bayesians, on the other hand, put their subjectivity on display and leave a hostage to fortune.

Initially, Bayesian analysis was restricted by limitations in computational power and it's only during the past two decades that advances in computer technology and software have permitted analysis of anything more than the simplest of problems. The complexity of the developments, however, is likely to prove inaccessible to most researchers.[5,74] This is important. Just as the problems associated with frequentist statistics have managed to escape detection in the medical research community because of their complexity, so, too, the mysteries of Bayesian analysis may hide a multitude of sins that will take a long time to surface.

It's well known that many people have difficulty in handling data presented in terms of conditional probabilities. By itself, this isn't an argument against Bayesian statistics although it may hinder attempts to gain widespread acceptance for this approach.

While the frequentist approach has been studied in depth and much has been written about the standards for the design, reporting and analysis of clinical trials, Bayesian statistics suffers from being less developed in the field of medical research. This is a considerable drawback.

Finally, as in the case of frequentist statisticians, Bayesians aren't free from internal squabbles. There are a number of different schools of Bayesian thinking[74] that are inconsistent with one another. Just as Fisher clashed with Neyman and Pearson, the different groups within Bayesian theory may become embroiled in protracted disputes.

Summary

The failings of frequentist statistics

More than a million clinical trials and epidemiological studies have been published over the last sixty years and, in almost every case, the statistical analysis has been based on frequentist methods. But the popularity of this approach hasn't been accompanied by a general understanding of what is involved, primarily because the concepts involved are far from straightforward. As Nickerson admitted,

> "The situation is not simple – it is confused and confusing – and a non-superficial understanding of the issues requires a considerable investment of time and effort... One finds conflicting opinions strongly held by knowledgeable people on various aspects of the topic, and it is not always easy to be sure of what one's own should be." [33]

The basic components of frequentist statistics lack clarity and transparency. They are slippery and illusive. It's difficult to feel at ease with them and, it seems, we just settle for accepting them uncritically. No wonder the many flaws have, for the most part, passed unnoticed.

When uncovered, however, these flaws provide the basis for a powerful attack on frequentist statistics and, in turn, on the conclusions of studies using these methods. Can we really trust the results of statistical analysis? In the light of the widespread criticism from authoritative voices in statistical circles and elsewhere in research, it would appear that, at the very least, we should treat frequentist methods with scepticism and be exceedingly circumspect in accepting the conclusions of epidemiological studies and large-scale RCTs based on conventional statistical analysis.

The promise of Bayesian statistics

In their vigorous and persistent criticisms of frequentist statistics, Bayesians have performed a valuable service. They, more than anyone else, have been responsible for challenging the status quo in research over recent times. Whether they will be successful in their attempts to overthrow the frequentists, however, remains uncertain.

The Bayesian alternative is interesting and appears to offer advantages. But it has its own problems. Whilst Bayesians promote priors as a valuable and indispensable part of statistical analysis in research, many neutral observers – not to mention the frequentists – don't share their enthusiasm. Moreover, the use of priors may, in practice, turn out to be more trouble than it's worth if, as suggested, it leads to intractable disputes about the choice of expert or the selection of background data on which to base prior distributions. And those waiting to be converted to Bayesian thinking may be reluctant to take the plunge in the absence of extensive experience with the new method in epidemiological studies and RCTs. They'll be wary of jumping prematurely. After all, they'll remember how the early promise of frequentist statistics was lost as, with the passage of time, more and more imperfections emerged. What's to say that Bayesian statistics won't meet the same fate?

In any case, the Bayesians would first have to usurp the frequentists which will be no easy matter. There would surely be a period of turmoil. Attention would be drawn to the frequentist failures creating a climate of extreme mistrust of statistics which would hardly be ideal for Bayesians. The slightest defect in their approach would be seized upon and marked as the beginning of the end of their brief reign.

Common failings of statistics-based research

Away from the statistical analysis, frequentists and Bayesians confront similar obstacles in medical research. All of the other problems related to internal validity and external validity apply to each method equally while the meaning of small differences to individuals is no less obscure with the Bayesian approach than with that of the frequentists.

As will be discussed in the following chapters, the absence of any reliable means of confirming the results of individual RCTs and the lack of any independent way of testing the statistical method in general present serious challenges to frequentists and Bayesians alike.

Lastly, questions about the basis of statistical causation apply to both approaches. The validity of the conclusions of statistics-based research depends on whether a small, statistically significant difference justifies causal inference. Yet, the closer this is examined, the less convincing it becomes.

References

1. Gigerenzer G, Krauss S, Vitouch O. The null ritual: what you always wanted to know about significance testing but were afraid to ask. In: Kaplan D (Ed.). The Sage Handbook of Quantitative Methodology for the Social Sciences. Sage, California. 2004; pp391-408.
2. Cohen LJ. An introduction to the philosophy of induction and probability. Oxford University Press. Oxford, 1989.
3. Spiegelhalter DJ, Myles JP, Jones DR, Abrams KR. An introduction to Bayesian methods in health technology assessment. BMJ 1999;319;508-12.
4. Lilford RJ, Braunholtz D. The statistical basis of public policy: a paradigm shift is overdue. BMJ 1996;313;603-7.
5. O'Hagan A, Luce BR. A primer on Bayesian statistics in health economics and outcomes research. Bayesian Initiative in Health Economics & Outcomes Research, Centre for Bayesian Statistics in Health Economics. Medtap International, Inc. 2003.
6. Fisher RA. Statistical Methods for Research Workers. Oliver and Boyd, 1925.
7. Fisher RA. The Design of Experiments. Oliver and Boyd, 1935.
8. Marks HM. Rigorous uncertainty: why RA Fisher is important. Int J Epidemiol 2003;32;932-7.
9. Armitage P. Fisher, Bradford Hill, and randomisation. Int J Epidemiol 2003;32;925-28.
10. Fisher RA. The arrangement of field experiments. Journal of the Ministry of Agriculture of Great Britain 1926;33;503-13.

11. Bodmer W. RA Fisher, statistician and geneticist extraordinary: a personal view. Int J Epidemiol 2003;32;938-42.
12. Neyman J, Pearson E. On the problem of the most efficient tests of statistical hypotheses. Philosophical Transactions of the Royal Society, Series A 1933;231;289-337.
13. Goodman SN. Toward evidence-based medical statistics. 1: The P value fallacy. Ann Intern Med 1999;130;995-1004.
14. Matthews RAJ. Facts versus factions: the use and abuse of subjectivity in scientific research. The European Science and Environment Forum. Working paper, September 1998.
15. Rozeboom WW. The fallacy of the null hypothesis significance test. Psychological Bulletin 1960;57;416-28.
16. Bakan D. The test of significance in psychological research. Psychological Bulletin 1966;66;423-7.
17. Yates F. Sir Ronald Fisher and the design of experiments. Biometrics 1964;20;307-21.
18. Lykken DT. Statistical significance in psychological research. Psychological Bulletin 1968;70;151-9.
19. Clark CA. Hypothesis testing in relation to statistical methodology. Review of Educational Research 1963;33;455-73.
20. Carver RP. The case against statistical significance testing. Harvard Educational Review 1978;48;378-399.
21. Cronbach LJ. Beyond the two disciplines of scientific psychology. American Psychologist 1975;30;116-27.
22. Cox DR. The role of significance tests. Scand J Stat 1977;4;49-70.
23. Evans SJ, Mills P, Dawson J. The end of the p value? Br Heart J 1988;60; 177-80.
24. Berger JO, Sellke T. Testing a point null hypothesis: the irreconcilability of P values and evidence. J Am Stat Assoc 1987;82;112-22.
25. Keuzenkamp HA, Magnus JR. On tests and significance in econometrics. Journal of Econometrics 1995;67;5-24.

26. Schmidt FL. Statistical significance testing and cumulative knowledge in psychology: implications for training of researchers. Psychological Methods 1996;1;115-129.
27. Cohen J. The earth is round (p>.05). American Psychologist 1994;49;997-1003.
28. Nester MR. An applied statistician's creed. Applied Statistics 1996;45; 401-10.
29. Greenwald AG, Gonzalez R, Harris RJ, Guthrie D. Effect sizes and p values: What should be reported and what should be replicated? Psychophysiology 1996;33;175-83.
30. Shaver JP. What statistical significance testing is, and what it is not. Journal of Experimental Education 1993;61;293-316.
31. Falk R, Greenbaum CW. Significance tests die hard: The amazing persistence of a probabilistic misconception. Theory and Psychology 1995;5;75-98.
32. Johnson DH. The insignificance of statistical significance testing. Journal of Wildlife Management 1999;63;763-72.
33. Nickerson RS. Null hypothesis significance testing: a review of an old and continuing controversy. Psychol Methods 2000;5;241-301.
34. Fidler F, Burgman MA, Cumming G et al. Impact of criticism of null-hypothesis significance testing on statistical reporting practices in conservation biology. Conservation Biology 2006;20;1539-44.
35. Loftus GR. On the tyranny of hypothesis testing in the social sciences. Contemporary Psychology 1991;36;102-5.
36. Rozeboom WW. Good science is not abductive, but hypothetico-deductive. In: Harlow LL, Mulaik SA, Steiger JH, Eds. *What if there were no significance tests?* Mahwah, NJ: Lawrence Erlbaum; 1997;335-39.
37. Thompson B. In praise of brilliance: Where praise really belongs. American Psychologist 1998;53;799-800.
38. Gigerenzer G. Reckoning with risk. The Penguin Press. London, 2002.
39. Oakes M. Statistical inference: A commentary for the social and behavioural sciences. Wiley, Chichester, UK. 1986.
40. Diamond GA, Forrester JS. Clinical trials and statistical verdicts: probable grounds for appeal. Ann Intern Med 1983;98;385-94.

41. Browner WS, Newman TB. Are all significant P values created equal? The analogy between diagnostic tests and clinical research. JAMA 1987;257; 2459-63.
42. Freeman PR. The role of P-values in analysing trial results. Stat Med 1993;12;1443-52.
43. Brophy JM, Joseph L. Placing trials in context using Bayesian analysis. GUSTO revisited by Reverend Bayes. JAMA 1995;273;871-5.
44. Berger JO, Berry DA. Statistical analysis and illusion of objectivity. American Scientist 1988;76;159-65.
45. Gliner JA, Leech NL, Morgan GA. Problems with null hypothesis significance testing (NHST): what do the textbooks say? The Journal of Experimental Education 2002;71;83-92.
46. Gibbons JD, Pratt JW. P-values: interpretation and methodology. American Statistician 1975;29;20-25.
47. Berkson J. Tests of significance considered as evidence. Journal of the American Statistical Association 1942;37;325-35.
48. Royall RM. The effect of sample size on the meaning of statistical tests. American Statistician 1986;40;313-5.
49. Brandt CL. Boen JR. A prevalent misconception about sample size, statistical significance and clinical importance. J Periodontol 1972;43;181-3.
50. Lindley DV. The analysis of experimental data: the appreciation of tea and wine. Teaching Statistics 1993;15;22-5.
51. Berkson J. Tests of significance considered as evidence. J Am Stat Assoc 1942;37;325-35.
52. Feinstein AR. P-values and confidence intervals: two sides of the same unsatisfactory coin. J Clin Epidemiol 1998;51;355-60.
53. Abelson RP. On the surprising longevity of flogged horses: Why there is a case for the significance test. Psychological Science 1997;8;12-5.
54. Cortina JM, Dunlap WP. On the logic and purpose of significance testing. Psychological Methods 1997;2;161-72.
55. Kirk RE. Practical significance: a concept whose time has come. Educational and Psychological Measurement 1996;56;746-59.

56. Glaser DN. The controversy of significance testing: misconceptions and alternatives. American Journal of Critical Care 1999;8;291-6.
57. Berkson J. Some difficulties of interpretation encountered in the application of the chi-square test. J Am Stat Assoc 1938;33;526-42.
58. Savage IR. Nonparametric statistics. J Am Stat Assoc 1957;52;331-344.
59. Johnson DH. Statistical sirens: the allure of nonparametrics. Ecology 1995;76;1998-2000.
60. Hagan RL. In praise of the null hypothesis statistical test. American Psychologist 1997;52;15-24.
61. Goodman SN. P values, hypothesis tests, and likelihood: implications for epidemiology of a neglected historical debate. Am J Epidemiol 1993;137; 485-96.
62. Lehman E. The Fisher, Neyman-Pearson theories of testing hypotheses: one theory or two? Journal of the American Statistical Association 1993;88; 1242-9.
63. Goodman SN. Multiple comparisons explained. Am J Epidemiol 1998;147; 807-12
64. Greenland S. Bayesian perspectives for epidemiological research: Foundations and basic methods. Int J Epidemiol 2006;35;765-775.
65. Meehl PE. Theory-testing in psychology and physics: A methodological paradox. Philosophy of Science 1967;34;103-115.
66. Nunnally JC. The place of statistics in psychology. Educational and Psychological Measurement 1960;20;641-50.
67. Binder A. Further considerations on testing the null hypothesis and the strategy and tactics of investigating theoretical models. Psychological Review 1963;70;107-15.
68. Edwards W. Tactical note on the relation between scientific and statistical hypotheses. Psychological Bulletin 1965;63;400-2.
69. Goodman SN. Toward evidence-based medical statistics. 2: The Bayes factor. Ann Intern Med 1999;130;1005-1013.
70. Marks HM. Trust and mistrust in the marketplace: statistics and clinical research 1945-60. Hist Sci 2000;38;343-55.

71. Porter TM. Trust in numbers: the pursuit of objectivity in science and public life. Princeton, NJ. Princeton University Press, 1995.
72. Freedman L. Bayesian statistical methods: Editorial. BMJ 1996;313;569-70.
73. Bayes T. *Essay Towards Solving a Problem in the Doctrine of Chances*, 1764.
74. Spiegelhalter DJ, Myles JP, Jones DR, Abrams KR. Bayesian methods in health technology assessment: a review. Health Technology Assessment 2000;Vol 4;No. 38.
75. Gill CJ, Sabin L, Schmid H. Why clinicians are natural bayesians. BMJ 2005;330;1080-3
76. Feinstein AR. Clinical Biostatistics XXXIX: The haze of Bayes, the aerial palaces of decision analysis, and the computerised Oijja board. Clin Pharmacol Ther 1977;21;482-96.
77. Lane N. Common sense, nonsense and statistics. J R Soc Med 1999;92; 202-5.

VII

Fraud in Medical Research

Fraud, in one form or another, is found in every walk of life. Politicians, bankers and hedge-fund managers commit fraud. So, too, do peers of the realm, senior police officers and judges. Football managers and famous comedians commit fraud. And many more humble individuals are similarly culpable when they complete their tax returns, fill in their monthly claims for expenses or apply for social security benefits.

It should come as no surprise, therefore, to learn that fraud occurs in medical research. The temptations are obvious. The lowly investigator can bolster his career prospects and achieve public acclaim, professors enhance their reputations and raise their chances of a knighthood, academic institutions gain prestige and attract funding, whilst pharmaceutical companies stand to make billions of dollars. We should expect fraud in medical research.

Setting the Scene

Fraud in science is nothing new. In *Betrayers of the Truth*,[1] Broad and Wade describe how research misconduct has occurred throughout history and provide endless examples to support their case. For instance, they describe how Ptolemy manufactured data in support of his theory that the earth was at the centre of the universe with the sun and planets revolving around it. But he wasn't alone. Many other illustrious scientists of the past were equally guilty.

There's a spectrum of offences that characterise research misconduct in science, ranging from plagiarism and minor manipulations of data at one end to complete fabrication of the results at the other. The more serious varieties are less common but the rewards are substantial. Needless to say, the temptations – at least for some individuals – are irresistible.

> "Science... is not an idealized interrogation of nature by dedicated servants of truth, but a human process governed by the ordinary human passions of ambition, pride, and greed, as well as by the well-hymned virtues attributed to men of science. But the step from greed to fraud is as small in science as in other walks of life." [1]

The frequency of fraud in scientific research is unknown but there are reasons to believe that it may be more common than is generally appreciated, especially if the more minor infringements are included. On the basis of their work, Broad and Wade suggest that fraud in science is far from being uncommon.[1]

Evidence of Fraud in Medical Research

- Individual case reports
- Information from government institutions (audits and reviews of legal cases)
- Surveys of those involved in research

The situation is no different in the sphere of medical research. However, as with obtaining accurate data about criminal activity in general, determining the frequency of fraud in medicine is no easy matter. If judged on the basis of cases proven in court, the frequency is bound to be underestimated. The situation is hardly improved by including all instances of fraud that appear in the medical or lay press, regardless of the outcome of legal proceedings. Individual cases provide conclusive proof that fraud occurs and also shed much light on the nature and circumstances of the offences but they tell us nothing of the magnitude of the problem.

Other sources, however, may enable more accurate estimates of the frequency of fraud in medical research. These include the work of government institutions and research studies by those with an interest in scientific fraud.

Examples of Fraud in Medical Research

For more than thirty years, instances of fraud in medical research have surfaced in the media. In the early 1970's, William Summerlin, an immunologist at the Sloan-Kettering Institute, claimed to have performed transplant experiments in animals.[1,2] Incredibly, the evidence for the successful skin graft from black to white mice was manufactured by colouring the skin of the white mice with a felt-tip pen. In the following decade, John Darsee at Harvard[1,2] and Robert Slutsky in San Diego[3] were each involved in separate instances of fraud in cardiology research culminating the retraction of numerous published papers and abstracts. Examples of fraud from the USA continue to appear in the literature. Eric Poehlman at the University of Vermont was sentenced to one year in jail in 2006 for multiple cases of data fabrication in publications about metabolic changes with ageing [4] while Luk Van Parijs of the Centre for Cancer Research at the Massachusetts Institute of Technology was fired for falsifying and fabricating research into immunological disease.[5]

Fraud, of course, isn't limited to the USA – indeed, their efforts to combat it have probably led to a false impression that it's more widespread in that country than elsewhere. It's ubiquitous. In South

Africa, for example, the results of two randomized trials of high-dose chemotherapy in breast cancer were later audited and found to be the product of research misconduct. Werner Bezwoda subsequently admitted fraud and the papers were retracted.[6] In Norway, Jon Sudbo published a completely fictitious study involving 454 patients which was reported to show that non-steroidal anti-inflammatory drugs reduced the risk of oral cancer.[7] In Holland, a neurologist was found guilty of fraud relating to the European Stoke Prevention Study (ESPC-2) after an inquiry showed that 90% of the patients audited hadn't participated in the trial.[8] And in South Korea, Hwang Woo-suk fabricated research claiming to have created the first stem cells from a cloned human embryo.[2]

In 2005, the *British Medical Journal* drew attention to the difficulties in proving conclusively that fraud has occurred.[9,10] Four years earlier, RK Chandra, working at the Memorial Hospital of Newfoundland, published a study claiming to show that vitamins and trace elements improved cognitive function in the elderly.[9] It was later alleged that the research was fabricated and this led to doubts about his previous 200 publications. Although the paper was retracted by the journal, the failure of the author to cooperate prevented any definite conclusion to the case.[9] A further example concerned a study by RB Singh purporting to show that the mortality following myocardial infarction was reduced by dietary treatment. Ever since its publication in 1992, the work had been viewed with suspicion, so much so that a review undertaken in 1995 recommended that the *BMJ* retract the paper. Yet, once again, after a refusal on the part of the author to provide data for further examination – he claimed that termites had destroyed the records – no final decision was possible.[10]

Fraud is certainly no stranger to the United Kingdom. An article in *The Observer* in 2003 documented five cases of general practitioners being involved in research misconduct.[11] Consultants, too, have been guilty of similar offences. AK Banerjee falsified data published in *Gut* in 1990. Samples claimed to have come from twelve healthy

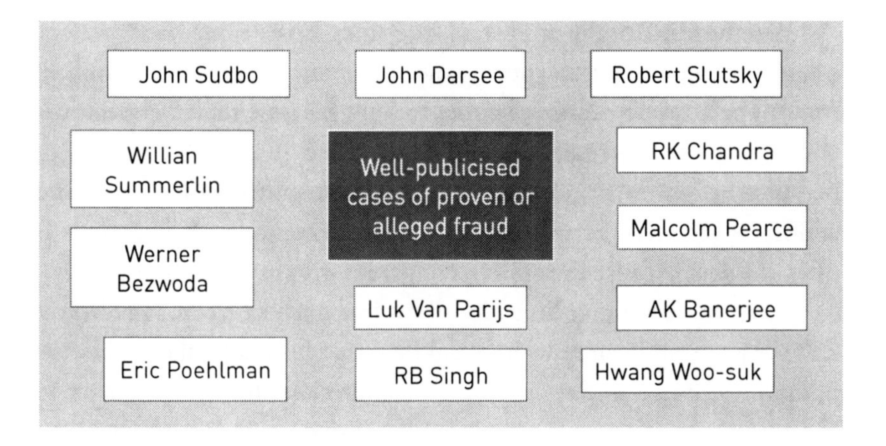

adults were, in fact, obtained from his own urine.[12] But perhaps the most well known case in recent times concerned Malcolm Pearce, an obstetrician and gynaecologist at St George's Hospital in London. In 1994, he published a paper claiming to have successfully re-implanted an ectopic pregnancy.[13] It turned out, however, that the patient never existed. That same year, he published the results of a randomised trial of gonadotrophin treatment for recurrent miscarriage in patients with polycystic ovarian syndrome.[14] But this study, too, was fraudulent and Pearce was removed from the medical register.[2]

Characteristic Features of Fraud in Medical Research

- Occur in prestigious academic institutions
- Exposed by whistle-blowers or suspicions of referees and editors
- A single instance often discloses multiple fraud in past publications
- Evidence of attempts at cover-up
- Difficulties in proving fraud

Whether in Britain or abroad, the story is the same. Researchers, often working in highly prestigious academic institutions, commit fraud. Their misdemeanours come to light because their behaviour is witnessed by fellow researchers – the so-called "whistle-blowers" – or because certain features of the data appear suspicious to referees and editors of journals. Frequently, a final judgement on their actions is often missing because they fail to cooperate with investigations.

Individual cases give little idea of the frequency of fraud. It's obvious that the problem is more widespread than that judged by the number of instances reported in the literature. To appreciate this, we only have to consider what occurs when a study is identified as fraudulent; the previous work of that individual, often published many years earlier, is then subjected to scrutiny and, in many cases, is found to contain evidence of past research misconduct. Without the discovery of fraud in the more recent research, the previous work would remain unchallenged in the medical literature.[9] Furthermore, there's evidence that when the question of fraud is raised, institutions to which the researchers belong attempt to cover up the matter to avoid adverse publicity. As Richard Smith commented,

> "Most cases are probably not publicised. They are simply not recognised, covered up altogether, or the guilty researcher is urged to retrain, move to another institution, or retire from research."[2]

There are, therefore, reasons to believe that the frequency of fraud is substantially underestimated when judged solely by the cases that reach the public domain.

Evidence of the Frequency of Fraud in Medical Research

Information collected by government institutions provides a guide to the frequency of fraud in medical research. For example, Shapiro and Charrow reviewed the data relating to 1,955 audits of clinical trials collected by the US Food and Drug Administration between 1977 and 1988.[15] They found that 12% of audits detected serious deficiencies between 1977 and 1985, decreasing to 7% for the period 1985-1988. Pownall, on the other hand, used information collected by the US Office of Research Integrity.[16] During the period 1993-1997, data on 1000 allegations of fraud were available and, of 150 cases formally investigated, 76 were shown to be due to research misconduct, mostly involving falsification (alteration of data), fabrication (inventing research) or plagiarism. However, findings like these clearly underestimate the size of the problem since they only take into account cases of fraud which have been reported to the authorities.

An alternative method for gauging the magnitude of the problem is to conduct surveys of those involved in medical research. Jacobsen and Halls sought the views of 152 principle investigators participating in clinical trials as identified from protocols submitted to ethics committees in Norway between 1986 and 1992.[17] The response rate to postal questionnaires was 70%. Eighteen percent of those who replied had been exposed to scientific misconduct and 27% knew of cases of fraud. The authors concluded that fraud in medicine is an increasing concern. Ramstam et al. surveyed 442 biostatisticians with a response rate of 37% and found that half were aware of fraudulent research projects.[18] Geggie, on the other hand, investigated clinicians by means of a questionnaire survey of newly appointed consultants in the Mersey Region between 1995 and 2000. Of 194 (64%) individuals who replied, 56% had observed some form of research misconduct while 6% admitted to being involved in fraud in medical research.[19]

More recent studies support the earlier findings. Gardner et al. surveyed 549 authors of clinical trials published between 1998 and 2001.[20] One percent of respondents reported that the paper in question misrepresented the research carried out, 5% said that fabrication had occurred in a study in which they had been involved in the previous ten years, while 17% knew of instances of research misconduct during the

Surveys of Researchers' Experience of Fraud

	Experience of fraud
Jacobsen & Halls (1995)17	27%
Ramstam et al. (2000)18	51%
Geggie (2001)19	56%
Gardner (2005)20	17%
Pryor et al. (2007)21	18%

last decade that hadn't been publicised. Similar results were reported by Pryor et al. in a survey of more than 5000 clinical researchers.[21] Although only about one-third responded to the questionnaire, 18% of these had first-hand experience of research misconduct.

Evidence from audits and surveys indicates that fraud in medical research is a much larger problem than suggested by the number of cases published in the media. This is certainly the view of commentators with a particular interest in research misconduct.[2,4,22]

The Trustworthiness of the Pharmaceutical Industry

For decades, reports of pharmaceutical companies being involved in dubious practices have appeared regularly in the lay press and the medical journals.

The pharmaceutical industry makes enormous profits from drugs shown to be effective in clinical trials. They're extensively involved in medical research and the evidence suggests that this has increased in recent times.[23,24] To a variable degree, they instigate and design the studies, select the centres and the investigators, participate in the collection and analysis of data, and influence the presentation and interpretation of the results. This, of course, doesn't prove that they commit fraud but it shows that they certainly have the motive, the opportunity and the means to do so.

There are, though, other aspects of the behaviour of the pharmaceutical industry that raise suspicions concerning their involvement with research fraud.

Sponsorship and the outcome of clinical trials

Numerous studies, including systematic reviews, have shown that clinical trials sponsored by the pharmaceutical industry tend to produce results more favourable to their products than do those which are independently funded.[25-31] The reasons for this finding are uncertain. Pharmaceutical companies clearly would be disinclined to publish research that casts doubt on the efficacy or safety of their products. They may also prematurely terminate trials that show unfavourable results in the early stages. And, of course, there's the tendency for journals not to publish research that has entirely negative findings. Studies that fail to show a therapeutic effect are more likely to be published if they are supported by government grants.[27,32] Thus, publication bias may be responsible, at least in part, for the association between industry-sponsored studies and favourable findings.

While clinical trials of poor quality are recognised to produce larger treatment effects than those meeting higher standards, meta-analyses suggest that there's no difference in methodological quality between industry-funded and independent studies.[26] However, the assessment of quality is not comprehensive and fails to exclude factors that may affect the outcome of trials.[33,34] Large-scale RCTs are so complicated that we can never be sure either that their results are entirely free from bias or that bias, if present, wasn't introduced deliberately to further the interests of a pharmaceutical company.

Manipulation of results of RCTs

Pharmaceutical companies that fund clinical research have ample opportunities to ensure that the results are presented in the most favourable light for their products. These include both the composition of the paper and the subsequent use of data from the publication in promotional material.

Given the size and complexity of publications of clinical trials, most readers focus on the abstract and the conclusions, and skim over – or omit entirely – the main body of the paper including the methods, the results and the discussion. Thus, they're unlikely to detect the distorted reporting and unwarranted conclusions that appear in medical journals, often on the instructions of the sponsors. Data manipulation, of course, is of equal concern in promotional material provided by pharmaceutical companies.[33,35,36]

Exaggerated claims about the benefits of medication are found throughout the literature reporting clinical research.[37] As discussed in chapter V, the use of relative risk reductions to inflate the beneficial effects is widespread in publications and promotional materials. We have already seen in chapter IV how the reporting of subgroup analysis is often deliberately selective in order to benefit the sponsor's product. And frankly misleading statements are no stranger to large-scale RCTs.[38] These are only some of the many ways in which the results may be manipulated.

Investigators coerced by the pharmaceutical industry

Unfortunately, it's not difficult to find instances of the pharmaceutical industry attempting to interfere with the publication of unfavourable research.[39-45] A survey of 306 senior executives from drug companies showed that 56% believed that industry prevented the publication of research carried out in universities.[41]

Careers have been damaged when the outcome of a study was not to the liking of its sponsor. The case of Nancy Olivieri well illustrates this point. While studying deferiprone – a drug believed to prevent iron accumulation in patients with haemoglobinopathies – she found that it failed to show benefit and might even worsen the development of hepatic fibrosis. Her results prompted action by the pharmaceutical company to prevent publication of the study. Later, she was subjected to lawsuits, was dismissed from her job at the Hospital for Sick Children in Toronto, and was charged with research misconduct. Allegations against her were eventually dismissed and the study was finally published.[46]

Other instances of similar coercion by pharmaceutical companies have occurred and are well documented in a review by Ahmer et al.[47]

Tales of disreputable practice by the pharmaceutical industry

To many, the pharmaceutical industry is the provider of medicines that alleviate suffering and prolong lives. To academic institutions, it's a major source of funding. To individual researchers, it supplies the finance that allows them to pursue their careers. And to the government, it's an important part of the Britain's economy, providing employment for a large number of people at home and earning vast sums overseas. It is, though, easy to forget that it's profit, not the desire to help mankind, that drives the pharmaceutical industry. Ultimately, companies will do whatever it takes to maximise their profits and this includes unethical or illegal activity. In the process, they endanger the lives of patients.

Examples of the pharmaceutical industry indulging in research misconduct are numerous.[47] The use of selective serotonin reuptake inhibitors for the treatment of depression has been the subject of much controversy. By failing to publish unfavourable results and by selectively reporting data – in particular, preferring per-protocol analysis to intention-to-treat analysis – pharmaceutical companies created a view of SSRIs as being more effective and less dangerous that is actually the case.[48,49] Their actions protected their products at the cost of the health of patients. The same may be said in the case of Vioxx. The company, Merck, Sharp and Dohme, withdrew the drug in 2004 yet they knew of the serious cardiovascular side-effects four years earlier and had deliberately concealed the data.[50] The list is endless. But one example, more than any other, illustrates the lengths to which pharmaceutical companies will go to defend their profits.

In the 1980's, Peter Wilmshurst came into conflict with a pharmaceutical company. The affair subsequently brought the industry into disrepute.[45] While studying the effects of amrinone on the heart, he found that, contrary to the expectations of the manufacturers, the drug had no positive inotropic action and, furthermore, produced frequent adverse events including thrombocytopoenia in up to half of the patients treated.[51]

What followed, according to Wilmshurst's account,[45] was an appalling series of actions on the part of Sterling-Winthrop. At first, the company requested the exclusion of patients who had shown a reduction in myocardial contractility from the analysis of the trial data. That would have had the effect of reversing the findings of the study and, hence, would have been research fraud. When the authors refused, they were threatened with litigation if they proceeded with publication. Then, attempts were made to discredit their work which included accusing them of fabricating data. Elsewhere, Sterling-Winthrop were ensuring that the results of other studies failed to reach the public domain. A professor in the USA, who was a consultant to the company, persuaded researchers not to publish unfavourable data relating to amrinone. While in Europe, Sterling-Winthrop submitted falsified data about the safety of the drug to the Netherlands Committee for the Evaluation of Medicines.[45]

Wilmshurst also drew attention to other aspects of the amrinone affair.[45] The original paper reporting possible benefits from the drug in 1978 claimed that all five authors were employed by Harvard Medical School when four were either employed by, or consultants to, Sterling-

Winthrop. Shortly afterwards, the company tried to suppress a report about the side-effects of amrinone. Wilmshurst also discovered that the drug didn't have a Clinical Trial Certificate – the five centres studying amrinone had been mislead by the company into believing that the required certification had been obtained. Apparently, the company threatened to withdraw its manufacturing from the United Kingdom if they were prosecuted for this offence against the Medicines Act. Eventually, Sterling-Winthrop conceded that amrinone was unsafe and withdrew the drug from the market in 1984.[45]

Wilmshurst's account is damning.[45] The pharmaceutical company involved stands accused of a failed attempt to persuade researchers to falsify data, bullying and intimidating researchers with threats of litigation, falsely accusing researchers of data fabrication, using academics with financial ties to the company to prevent publication of studies, falsifying safety data submitted to regulatory authorities, concealing the nature of the employment of authors in a published paper and performing clinical trials on a drug without a license. It reads like an inventory of offences in medical research.

The Wilmshurst Affair

Actions of the pharmaceutical company

- Persuading researchers to falsify data
- Bullying and intimidating researchers
- Preventing publication of other related studies
- Falsifying safety data for regulatory authorities
- Concealing conflicts of interest of authors
- Performing clinical trials without a licence for the drug

But is this just an isolated instance? Is this particular company simply a bad apple in a barrel of otherwise good ones? There seems to be no reason to believe that this is the case. Pharmaceutical companies compete against one another in the same market. Staff are recruited from the same pool of applicants and move freely among the various companies from one job to another. They have the same pressures to succeed and the same penalties for failure. Why, then, shouldn't they share the same propensity to commit research fraud when the situation demands?

The problem is that, until there are more individuals with the courage and tenacity of Peter Wilmshurst, we will simply not know the extent of research fraud perpetrated by the pharmaceutical industry.

Conclusions

Fraud occurs in medical research and, although accurate estimates of its frequency aren't available, there are reasons to believe that it's far more common than previously thought.

No one should be surprised. The rewards to individuals and to institutions carrying out research are considerable and there are enough examples to show that time and again the temptations have proved to be irresistible. Perhaps, though, the greatest concern is the involvement of the pharmaceutical industry in medical research. Too often in the past, it has indulged in disreputable practices in the pursuit of profit. Yet still it's allowed to be intimately involved in medical research. Its supporters argue that an independent steering committee and other subcommittees protect studies against interference. But we must treat the independence of the members of the steering committee with a good deal of scepticism – the influence of the pharmaceutical industry is, after all, widespread. In any case, even if those charged with the responsibility for overseeing clinical research were whiter than white, they would still not be able to ensure that fraud is eradicated from medical research.

But rewards, by themselves, are insufficient to account for fraud in medical research. Intelligent individuals weigh up the benefits and the risks, and a crucial part of this calculation is their assessment of the chances of being caught and punished. That they pursue their chosen course shows that they judge the probability of being found out to be low. The evidence suggests that they're correct. Moreover, even if fraud is uncovered, there's no guarantee that it will be taken further. History repeatedly shows that academic institutions are slow to take action and, when they do so, often embark upon a cover-up to prevent adverse publicity.

In the case of epidemiological studies and large RCTs, there are other reasons to believe that fraud will remain secret. The complexity of these studies and the frequent poor reporting hide a multitude of sins. But the main obstacle to identifying fraud is the lack of any means to confirm or refute the results of this type of research. This is a fundamental failing of statistics-based medical research. It militates against the discovery of falsified or fabricated data and allows those who have perpetrated fraud to sleep soundly at night.

References

1. Broad W, Wade N. Betrayers of the Truth. Oxford University Press. Oxford, England. 1985.
2. Smith R. Research misconduct: the poisoning of the well. J R Soc Med 2006;99;232-7.
3. Petersdorf RG. The pathogenesis of fraud in medical science. Ann Intern Med 1986;104;252-4.
4. Sheehan JG. Fraud, conflict of interest, and other enforcement issues in clinical research. Cleveland Clinic Journal of Medicine 2007;74(suppl 2);S63-67.
5. Reich ES. Bad data fail to halt patients. Nature 2006;439;379.

6. Weiss RW, Gill GG, Hudis CA. An on-site audit of the South African trial of high-dose chemotherapy for metastatic breast cancer and associated publications. J Clin Oncol 2001;19;2771-7.
7. Eaton L. Norwegian researcher admits that his data were faked. BMJ 2006;332;193.
8. Hoeksema HL, Troost J, Grobbee DE, Wiersinga WM, et al. A case of fraud in a neurological pharmaceutical trial. Ned Tijdschr Geneeskd 2003;147;1372-7.
9. Smith R. Investigating the previous studies of a fraudulent author. BMJ 2005;331;288-91.
10. White C. Suspected research fraud: difficulties of getting at the truth. BMJ 2005;331;281-8.
11. Barnett A. Patients used as drug 'guinea pigs'. *The Observer*, Sunday February 9th 2003.
12. Ferriman A. Consultant suspended for research fraud. BMJ 2000;321; 1429.
13. Pearce JM, Manyonda IT, Chamberlain GVP. Term delivery after intrauterine relocation of an ectopic pregnancy. Br J Obs Gynaecol 1994;101;716-7.
14. Pearce JM, Hamid RI. Randomised controlled trial of the use of human chorionic gonadotrophin in recurrent miscarriage associated with polycystic ovaries. Br J Obs Gynaecol 1994;101;685-8.
15. Shapiro MF, Charrow RP. The role of data audits in detecting scientific misconduct. Results of FDA program. JAMA 1989;261; 2505-11.
16. Pownall M. Falsifying data is main problem in US research fraud review. BMJ 1999;318;1164.
17. Jacobsen G, Hals A. Medical investigators' views about ethics and fraud in medical research. J R Coll Physicians Lond. 1995;29;405-9.
18. Ranstam J, Buyse M, George SL, et al. Fraud in medical research: an international survey of biostatisticians. ISCB Subcommittee on Fraud. Control Clin Trials 2000;21;415-27.
19. Geggie D. A survey of newly appointed consultants' attitudes towards research fraud. J Med Ethics 2001;27;344-6.

20. Gardner W, Lidz CW, Hartwig KC. Authors' reports about research integrity problems in clinical trials. Contemp Clin Trials. 2005;26;244-51.
21. Pryor ER, Habermann B, Broome ME. Scientific misconduct from the perspective of research coordinators: a national survey. J Med Ethics 2007;33;365-9.
22. Lock S, Wells F., Eds. Fraud and Misconduct in Medical Research. 2nd Edition. London, UK. BMJ Publishing Group, 1996.
23. Anderson JJ, Felson DT, Meenan RF. Secular changes in published clinical trials of second-line agents in rheumatoid arthritis. Arthritis Rheum 1991;34;1304-9.
24. Dorman PJ, Counsell C, Sandercock PA. Reports of randomised trials in acute stroke, 1955-1995: what proportions were commercially sponsored? Stroke 1999;30;1995-8.
25. Bekelman JE, Li Y, Gross CP. Scope and impact of financial conflicts of interest in biomedical research: a systematic review. JAMA 2003;289;454-65.
26. Lexchin J, Bero LA, Djulbegovic B, Clark O. Pharmaceutical industry sponsorship and research outcome and quality: systematic review. BMJ 2003;326;1167-70.
27. Yaphe J, Edman R, Knishkowy B, Herman J. The association between funding by commercial interests and study outcome in randomized controlled drug trials. Family Practice 2001;18;565-8.
28. Davidson RA. Source of funding and outcome in clinical trials. J Gen Intern Med 1986;1;155-8.
29. Cho MK, Bero LA. The quality of drug studies published in symposium proceedings. Ann Intern Med 1996;124;485-9.
30. Rochon PA, Gurwitz JH, Simms RW, et al. A study of manufacturer supported trials of non-steroidal anti-inflammatory drugs in the treatment of arthritis. Arch Intern Med 1994;154;157-63.
31. Ahmer S, Arya P, Anderson D, Faruqui R. Conflict of interest in psychiatry. Psychiatric Bulletin 2005;29;302-4.
32. Lexchin J. Is there a bias in industry supported clinical research? Can J Clin Pharmacol 1995;2;15-8.

33. Bero LA, Rennie D. Influences on the quality of published drug studies. Int J Technol Assess Health Care 1996;12;209-37.
34. Gotzsche P. Methodology and overt and hidden bias in reports of 196 double-blind trials of nonsteroidal anti-inflammatory drugs in rheumatoid arthritis. Control Clin Trials 1989;10;31-56.
35. Johansen HR, Gotzsche PC. Problems in the design and reporting of trials of antifungal agents encountered during meta-analysis. JAMA 1999;282; 1752-9.
36. Safer DJ. Design and reporting modifications in industry-sponsored comparative psychopharmacology trials. J Nerv Ment Dis 2002;190;583-92.
37. Penston J. Fiction and Fantasy in medical research: the large-scale randomised trial. The London Press. London, 2003. Chapter V.
38. Gruppo Italiano per lo Studio della Sopravvivenza nell'Infarcto Miocardico. GISSI-3: effects of lisinopril and transdermal glyceryl trinitrate singly and together on 6-week mortality and ventricular function after acute myocardial infarction. *Lancet* 1994;343;1115-22.
39. McCarthy M. Company sought to block paper's publication. Lancet 2000;356;1659.
40. Rennie D. Thyroid storm JAMA 1997;277;1238-43.
41. Blumenthal D, Causino N, Campbell E, Louis K. Relationships between academic institutions and industry in the life sciences - an industry survey. NEJM 1996;334;368-73.
42. Hailey D. Scientific harassment by pharmaceutical companies: time to stop. CMAJ 2000;162; 212-3.
43. Hemminki E, Hailey D, Koivusalo M. The courts – a challenge to health technology assessment. Science 1999;285;203-4.
44. Shuchman M. Drug firm threatens suit over MD's product review. Globe and Mail 1999; Nov 17;Sect A:5.
45. Wilmshurst P. Dishonesty in medical research. Med Leg J 2007;75;3-12.
46. Olivieri NF, Brittenham GM. Final results of the randomised trials of deferiprone and deferoxamine. Blood 1997;90(Suppl 1);264.
47. Ahmer S, Haider II, Anderson D, Arya P. Do pharmaceutical companies selectively report clinical trial data. Pak J Med Sci 2006;22;338-46.

48. Whittington CJ, Kendall T, Fonagy P, et al. Selective serotonin reuptake inhibitors in childhood depression: systematic review of published versus unpublished data. Lancet 2004;363;1341-5.
49. Melander H, Ahlqvist-Rastad J, Meijer G, Beerman B. Evidence b(i)ased medicine – selective reporting from studies sponsored by pharmaceutical industry: review of studies in new drug applications. BMJ 2003;326;1171-3.
50. Horton R. Vioxx, the implosion of Merck, and aftershocks at the FDA. Lancet 2004;364;1995-6.
51. Wilmshurst PT, Webb-Peploe MM. Side-effects of amrinone therapy. Br Heart J 1983;49;447-51.

VIII

Answering Doubting Thomas

Dubious internal validity... flawed external validity... queries about the statistical theory... worries about research fraud – it's enough to wreck the confidence of all but the most ardent supporters of statistics-based medicine.

When faced with a newly published epidemiological study or randomised controlled trial, how do we know whether the conclusion is valid? How do we know that a generalisation based on the data is true? How do we confirm or refute the claims of statistics-based research?

Wanting to test assertions about phenomena in the world around us isn't being paranoid. It's part of our nature. We ask for evidence; we ask for proof; and, in the normal course of events, our request for evidence is granted. Shane Warne tells someone who knows nothing about cricket that a leg-spin bowler is able to produce different deliveries, for example, the googly pitching and turning in the opposite direction to the standard leg-break. They don't believe him. He shows them. That's an example of providing convincing evidence. But, as we'll see, evidence to show that the conclusion of a RCT is valid isn't so readily forthcoming.

In this chapter, we'll examine whether or not it's possible to test the result of a particular epidemiological study or RCT. Then, more importantly, we'll turn our attention to the question of whether it's possible to test the method used in statistics-based research in general.

Testing the Evidence

Lessons from school

Performing experiments is a basic part of learning science in school. This enables the pupils to gain an early understanding of the scientific method. But it also allows them to test the claims made in their textbooks. They learn that they don't have to take the words of their teachers on trust.

For example, simple and easy to carry out experiments confirm the teachers' claims that opposite poles of magnets attract and similar poles repel each other, that iodine changes from brown to dark blue when it comes into contact with starch, and that alkalis neutralise acids. If the student questions something, it can be tested. He may not believe the teacher's assertions that adding cold water to anhydrous white copper sulphate changes it to blue hydrated copper sulphate and that the reaction is exothermic but this could easily be demonstrated. He would be able to see the colour change and feel the heat generated.

Subjects like physics, chemistry and biology involve causal generalisations that may be tested and the results are not only predictable but readily discernible to our senses.

Satisfying the doubters

We all have something of Doubting Thomas about us. Unless we're pathologically gullible, we don't take everything that we're told at face value. Instead, we ask for evidence.

Advertisers are well aware of this and have been using it to their advantage for decades. We remember the grainy black and white images comparing the whiteness of shirts, sheets or towels – proof that Daz, Omo or Persil washes whiter than ordinary brands. Similarly, we're familiar with the endlessly long parallel tables laden with crockery and cutlery that show that Fairy liquid is superior to standard washing-up detergents. And the same technique has been used with everything from toothpaste to acne lotions.

Perhaps the best example from the world of television adverts was the Duracell rabbit. It had all of the features of a controlled experiment. It began with a platoon of identical, drum-playing toy rabbits across the screen. The only difference between them was the source of the energy for their electric motors. Gradually, those supplied with ordinary batteries fell silent leaving the Duracell rabbit to continue drumming on and on. The message was clear: Duracell batteries last longer than ordinary ones.

Of course, we may doubt the truth of the so-called evidence – especially in the case of the whiter-than-white claims of soap powder manufacturers. But this doesn't detract from the significance of the advertisers' decision to market the products in this way. They know only too well our tendency to ask for proof and our natural inclination to believe what's before our eyes. They also know that we're convinced by evidence in the form of a simple experiment – when we're shown what happens in the absence and in the presence of the cause.

Scientific experiments

The history of science is marked by astonishingly original experiments. Often they're very simple. Isaac Newton's experiment on light refraction is a prime example. He demonstrated that white light is broken up into its constituent colours by passing through a glass prism and that the spectrum of coloured light produced is reconstituted into white light by passage through a further prism. Were anyone to doubt this phenomenon, he would be shown the error of his ways by repeating the original experiment. Indeed, millions of students have done precisely this and Newton's findings have always been confirmed. Humphrey Davey's experiments with electrolysis and those of Francois-Marie

Raoult to show the effect of solutes on the freezing point of water are also regularly performed in schools and universities, again with consistent results. The list is endless and, in each case, the outcome is always predictable. In other words, these experiments lead directly to universal generalisations.

This raises a crucial issue. If a scientific claim is presented in terms of a universal generalisation, then it applies to all cases of the phenomenon. For example, the generalisation that adding sodium chloride to water lowers its freezing point entails that whenever the experiment is performed, the outcome will be the same. Thus, the original experiment may be replicated. This is the ultimate test of the result of an experiment and of the generalisation derived from it.

Palpable evidence

Replication isn't only a cardinal feature of the scientific method but it has an important role in showing that a causal claim is true. In other words, it's not just a matter of knowing that replication has been carried out and that the results were the same as those of the original experiment; it offers something more – the opportunity for us to see an example of this particular cause and effect relationship in action. We're persuaded by witnessing such things.

It's the possibility of demonstrating the causal phenomenon that holds so much weight in convincing others of the truth of a scientific generalisation. There are few better examples than that which occurred during the Presidential Commission into the cause of the space shuttle Challenger accident in 1986.[1] For some time, interest was focussed on the O-ring seals. The launch that ended in disaster took place on a particularly cold morning and, reasonably, it was argued that the low temperatures had affected the properties of the O-ring seal on the rocket boosters. However, by the time the Commission began, there was no agreement on this issue.

In the midst of the proceedings, Richard Feynman, a renowned physicist, asked for a glass of iced water. Then, he took a piece of the O-ring material held in a small clamp and immersed it in the water. On cooling, the material lost its ability to return to its original shape when the clamp was removed.

> "I took this stuff that I got out of your seal and I put it in ice water, and I discovered that when you put some pressure on it for a while and then undo it, it doesn't stretch back. It stays the same dimension. In other words, for a few seconds at least and more seconds than that, there is no resilience in this particular material when it is at a temperature of 32 degrees." [1]

A simple experiment using a small piece of an O-ring, a metal clamp and a glass of iced water provided strong evidence that the temperature on the day of the launch of the shuttle was sufficient to impair the proper functioning of the O-ring seals and that this led directly to the explosion. But why did those present find this to be so convincing? Why did Feyman's experiment seem to trump all the written and oral evidence given to the Commission? The point is, of course, that it was a practical demonstration. In a textbook, the assertion that lowering the temperature alters the properties of the O-ring material is one thing; seeing the effect of lowering the temperature on the properties of the O-ring material is quite another.

Testing the Results of Statistics-Based Research

Unlike the physical sciences which produce universal generalisations, statistics deals only with particular generalisations.[2] In other words, a generalisation derived from statistical studies applies only to *some* members of the reference class and these members are anonymous. Statistics-based research can never produce anything other than particular generalisations because it's used precisely in the situation where the reference class is heterogeneous with respect to the outcome. In both the placebo and drug groups, only some individuals will develop the outcome and, of those receiving active treatment, only some will have the outcome prevented by the drug under investigation.

It's the use of such mixtures of individuals with different characteristics relevant to the outcome that is both the reason for choosing statistics-based research and the source of the problems in testing the results of these studies.

Testing the Results of RCTs

- Evidence from single cases
- Evidence from clinical practice with multiple cases
- Evidence from epidemiological studies
- Evidence from other RCTs

Evidence derived from single cases

The validity of a generalisation based on statistical research can't be tested by observing the phenomenon in a single case. Consider, for example, a large study that showed 5% of patients receiving placebo died compared with 4% of those given the active drug over a period of five years. This entails that the drug is of no possible benefit in terms of survival to 95% of patients. In the subgroup of 5% who would have died without treatment, one-fifth will survive if given the drug. It follows that, if we observe any individual who survives five years, we can't assume that this is an instance of treatment success. In fact, it's much more likely that they'd have survived regardless of treatment.

Thus we can't, in principle, observe an instance of treatment success. We can, though, observe treatment failure. Any instance of a patient developing the outcome whilst taking the drug is unequivocal evidence of therapeutic failure. It says a great deal about the statistical approach to medical research that it leads to the situation in which we are able to experience instances of treatment failure but never of treatment success.

Evidence from multiple cases

While the single case is of no value in confirming or refuting the results of large RCTs, perhaps everyday clinical experience would be a better alternative. Physicians and surgeons with a special interest are often in the position of caring for hundreds of patients with a particular disease and this would seem to be an opportunity to compare the outcome of particular treatments with the results of published studies. But, on closer inspection, this would be equally unsuccessful. How would they know that there were no differences between their patients and those in the studies? For example, how could they be sure that their sample wasn't biased in favour of those with better outcomes? More importantly, there would be no randomisation and no controls.

As soon as we think about comparing observational data derived from clinical practice with the results of RCTs, we realise that it's futile. In any case, the numbers of patients required to confirm or refute the small differences detected in the large-scale studies wouldn't be available. Put another way, the decision to investigate small differences protects the results of large-scale studies from any challenge based on clinical experience.

As in the case of a single instance, evidence from the observation of multiple patients would never permit any reliable inference about the treatment effect. Thus, personal experiences can play no role in testing the results of large-scale studies based on statistics.

Evidence from epidemiological studies

Nowadays, it's not uncommon to encounter epidemiological studies claiming to support the results of large RCTs. Data-bases of diseases and those of drug prescribing may be combined to investigate the different clinical outcomes in patients receiving a drug and those left untreated. The ease and speed with which such studies may be performed and analysed has led to a proliferation of epidemiological data relating to drug efficacy.

A typical example of such studies was published in 2008.[3] As stated in the title, the study claimed to be a "replication of the Scandinavian Simvastatin Survival Study". Using the General Practice Research Database (GPRD) in the United Kingdom, a cohort study was carried out to compare the cardiovascular outcomes in patients treated with statins and those not receiving the drugs. A single sentence in the abstract, however, exposes the weaknesses of the research: "All aspects of the RCT except randomisation were replicated to the extent possible in the GPRD study."[3]

Epidemiological data are of little use in testing the results of RCTs. As has been noted repeatedly, observational studies are widely considered to be less reliable than large randomised trials. It follows, therefore, that any dispute about the findings of clinical trials and those of observational studies would be settled in favour of those using intervention and randomisation. But, if epidemiological studies can't challenge RCTs, then neither can they confirm the findings. When it comes to testing the results of RCTs, epidemiological studies are redundant.

Replication of RCTs

If we question the results of a RCT, it may be thought that the issue would be settled by replicating the trial, just as is done in science. But it's not possible to re-create the exact conditions of the original study.

While the conduct of a clinical trial, the selection of patients and the treatment regimens are specified in the protocol, it would be a mistake to assume that the descriptions of each were exhaustive. Many elements are unspecified or vague; many others are taken for granted and omitted altogether. In particular, the selection criteria for patient participation aren't sufficient to enable the recruitment of a sample that closely resembles the original study population. There'll always be differences between the characteristics of patients in different studies.

But even if it were possible to describe every detail in the protocol with the utmost precision, it's unlikely that conditions identical to those in the original trial could be reproduced. Large-scale RCTs are often long-term enterprises and it's not exceptional for more than ten years to elapse between the decision to design a study and its eventual publication. In that time, there'll be many developments in medicine: new drugs will become available, new surgical techniques will appear and indications for treatment will be adjusted; new diagnostic tests will be introduced that change the definition of the disease; and advances in our understanding of the underlying pathological processes will influence how we manage the patients.

But we mustn't forget the role of investigators. They interpret the protocol and make day-to-day decisions about the care of patients. Thus, their education, experience and skill affect the conduct and outcome of the trials. However, these features also change over time. In any case, given the rapid turnover of staff, it's highly unlikely that the same investigators would be available if replication were to be attempted.

It's not just the insurmountable difficulties in re-creating the same conditions as were present in the original trial. It's also the fact that there's no incentive to attempt replication. If a RCT has shown a therapeutic benefit from a drug, it wouldn't be in the interest of the sponsoring pharmaceutical company to repeat it. They'd have nothing to gain and everything to lose if the second study failed to confirm the effect. There's little incentive, either, for government funded institutions to support replication, particularly in view of the high costs of such trials.

When the Results of RCTs Collide

The difficulties involved with the idea that one RCT may confirm or refute the results of another are clearly seen in the case of two very similar studies published in 2003 and 2004 that produced conflicting results.

EUROPA

The purpose of the EUROPA study was to determine the effect of perindopril, an ACE inhibitor, on the occurrence of cardiovascular events in patients with stable ischaemic heart disease.[4] A multi-centre, randomised, double-blind, placebo-controlled trial was performed in 23 countries in Europe. Between 1997 and 2000, 12,218 patients were randomised to receive either perindopril or placebo and followed up for an average of 4.2 years. The primary outcome was a composite of cardiovascular death, non-fatal myocardial infarction or cardiac arrest with successful resuscitation.

The results, published in 2003, showed statistically significant reductions in the primary endpoint and myocardial infarction but no reduction was observed in either cardiovascular deaths or overall mortality. The findings were used to support the recommendation that all patients with ischaemic heart disease should be given ACE inhibitors.[4]

EUROPA Study

	Perindopril	Placebo	Relative risk reduction	P-value
Primary endpoint	8.0%	9.9%	20%	0.0003
Myocardial infarction	4.8%	6.2%	22%	0.001
Cardiovascular mortality	3.5%	4.1%	14%	0.107
Total mortality	6.1%	6.9%	11%	0.1

Problems with EUROPA

1. The original primary end-point was a composite of cardiovascular mortality, non-fatal myocardial infarction, unstable angina and cardiac arrest. This was changed in 2002, two years after the end of patient recruitment and one year before the end of data collection. In addition, the duration of the trial was extended by one year. The reasons for changing the protocol were claimed to be the introduction of new methods for the diagnosis of myocardial infarction and the relatively low mortality from cardiovascular disease. The authors stated that the decision to alter the protocol was taken by the EUROPA steering committee without knowledge of the data analysis.[4]
2. Initially, 13,655 patients were registered but 1437 (10.5%) were excluded following a run-in phase of treatment with perindopril for up to four weeks. Most of the patients were excluded for reasons related to treatment with the ACE inhibitor – for example, hypotension, raised creatinine, hyperkalaemia, other adverse drug reactions or poor compliance.
3. The rate of drop-outs and withdrawals following randomisation was high – 23% in the perindopril group compared with 21% of those receiving placebo. Furthermore, 13% of patients declined to continue with the extended period of observation and were withdrawn. The reporting in the paper on these issues is unclear.
4. All five members of the EUROPA executive committee declared a conflict of interest in respect of honoraria or research grants received from the pharmaceutical company sponsoring the study.[4]

PEACE

The PEACE study was also designed to determine the effect of ACE inhibitors on the occurrence of cardiovascular events in patients with stable ischaemic heart disease.[5] A multi-centre, randomised, double-blind, placebo-controlled trial was performed in the USA, Puerto Rico, Canada and Italy. Between 1996 and 2000, a total of 8,290 patients were randomised to treatment with trandolapril or placebo for an average of 4.8 years. The primary endpoint was a composite of cardiovascular death, myocardial infarction or coronary revascularisation.

PEACE Study

	Trandolapril	Placebo	Relative risk reduction	P-value
Primary endpoint	21.9%	22.5%	4%	0.43
Myocardial infarction	5.3%	5.3%	0%	1.0
Cardiovascular mortality	3.5%	3.7%	5%	0.67
Total mortality	7.2%	8.1%	11%	0.13

In contrast to the earlier trial, the PEACE study failed to show any difference in the primary end-point between the active drug and placebo. Nor, for that matter, were any treatment effects noted in the case of the secondary endpoints including myocardial infarction, cardiovascular deaths and total mortality.[5]

Problems with PEACE

1. The original primary end-point specified in the study protocol was a composite of cardiovascular mortality or non-fatal myocardial infarction. However, one year after the trial began, it was apparent that the intended recruitment of 14,100 patients would not be achieved. In 1997, the sample size was almost halved and the primary end-point was changed to a composite of cardiovascular mortality, non-fatal myocardial infarction or coronary revascularisation.

Again, the authors claimed that this decision was made without knowledge of the data collected at the time.[5]

2. The PEACE study also included a run-in phase in which patients received trandolapril for two weeks and were subsequently excluded if they were poorly compliant with medication or developed adverse drug reactions including hyperkalaemia, raised creatinine and hypotension. The number of patients excluded because of the outcome of the run-in phase was not provided.
3. The study was sponsored by pharmaceutical companies. Members of the executive committee, steering committee and the writing committee admitted to conflicts of interest in respect of lecture fees and research grants from the pharmaceutical industry.[5]

Thus, we have two similar RCTs, published within a year of each other, producing very different results. What, then, is to be said about the conflicting findings? More specifically, do the results of PEACE refute those of EUROPA?

The arguments proposed to account for the conflicting results

In their discussion section, the authors of the PEACE study were keen to avoid any conflict.[5] In fact, they went out of their way to account for the differences between the results of PEACE and EUROPA by proposing that the patients in the studies were different. They argued that the characteristics of the two samples of patients differed in respect of blood pressure, cholesterol and creatinine levels, left ventricular function and the frequency of previous revascularisation procedures. This, they claimed, resulted in the patients in the PEACE study being at less risk of cardiovascular events than those in EUROPA.[5] Others, however, disagree that these differences explain the failure of the PEACE study to replicate the findings of EUROPA.[6]

Baseline Differences

	EUROPA	PEACE
Age (mean)	60yrs	64yrs
Females	15%	18%
Previous ischaemic heart disease		
Myocardial infarction	65%	55%
Percutaneous intervention	29%	41%
Coronary artery bypass	29%	39%
Previous vascular disease		
Strokes/TIAs	3%	6%
Diabetes	12%	17%
Hypertension	27%	45%
Medication		
Anti-platelet drugs	92%	90%
Beta-blockers	61%	60%
Lipid-lowering drugs	57%	70%
Blood pressure		
Systolic mmHg (mean)	137	134
Diastolic mmHg (mean)	82	78

Examining the baseline data of each RCT, it would also appear that the authors of the PEACE study were being biased in selecting those features that supported their case. They might just as easily have commented on the features that would tend to make their own group of patients at increased risk of future cardiovascular events – for example, they were older and had a higher prevalence of previous cerebrovascular disease, diabetes and hypertension – compared with those in the EUROPA study. It's also noticeable that no mention was given to the fact that the studies were performed in different locations – EUROPA entirely in Europe, PEACE mostly in North America. No doubt, the pharmaceutical companies manufacturing ACE inhibitors were anxious to keep this quiet – showing that these drugs weren't so effective in the USA would damage their market.

Interestingly, the title of both papers refers to patients with "stable coronary heart disease" and this term is repeated in the text.[4,5] Furthermore, the authors of each paper also use the term "low-risk" to describe the patients recruited. Yet, despite this, it's argued that the groups are different in respect of the outcomes. If this is the case, it would suggest that their ability to identify patients at low risk is poor.

Other commentators have proposed, for example, that different ACE inhibitors have different pharmacological properties including bioavailability and penetration into atherosclerotic plaques, and that the trials differed in terms of the therapeutic regimens as well as in the proportion of patients reaching the target dose of the drug.[6] These have the flavour of ad hoc explanations.

Direct Comparison of EUROPA and PEACE Studies

	Primary Endpoint*	Relative risk reduction	P-value
EUROPA			
Perindopril	8.0%		
Placebo	9.9%	20%	0.0003
PEACE			
Trandolapril	8.3%		
Placebo	8.6%	4%	0.62

* Common primary end-point of cardiovascular mortality or myocardial infarction or cardiac arrest as used in the EUROPA study

Understandably, differences in outcome have been attributed to differences in the primary end-point between the two studies. The authors of PEACE specifically addressed this problem in the discussion section where they re-calculated their own data in terms of the end-point used in EUROPA.[5] It made no difference; using the new composite endpoint failed to alter the conclusions of PEACE.

Perhaps, strangest of all, is the suggestion that PEACE was inadequately powered to detect statistical differences.[6] This cannot be accepted. It wasn't a case of the differences between the groups in respect of the various end-points not reaching statistical significance; there were no differences. The primary end-point, the proportion of patients with myocardial infarction and the cardiovascular mortality were the same in patients given trandolapril as they were in the placebo group.

Lessons from EUROPA and PEACE

The EUROPA and PEACE studies are typical examples of modern day large-scale randomised trials. In each case, many thousands of patients were recruited because it was expected that the difference in primary end-point would be small. Furthermore, composite primary end-points were used in both studies so that sufficient numbers of events would be observed, thus assisting in the detection of statistically significant differences.

All of the criticisms made about RCTs in previous chapters apply equally to both EUROPA and PEACE. In addition, however, there are specific problems raised by these studies in relation to the way in which the conflicting data were handled.

a) *Internal validity*: Whether or not the conditions for internal validity were satisfied is unclear. We know nothing, for example, about the success of blinding during the either EUROPA or PEACE, and the number of withdrawals and drop-outs in each study was considerable.

b) *Change of protocol*: What we do know is that changes were made to the protocol of both studies after the data collection had started. As noted by the authors of EUROPA, such action is unusual. Moreover, it clearly threatens the internal validity. Although it's claimed that the decision to change the protocol was taken without knowledge of the data collected at that time, this has to be taken on trust.

c) *External validity*: Given the arguments about the importance of demographic factors in explaining the conflicting results, it's difficult to say anything meaningful about the generalisability of the conclusions. One minute the patients recruited to EUROPA are at low risk, the next – when PEACE is published – they're at not at low risk, at least as specified in the later RCT. The intention of each study was to recruit low risk patients but it seems that the criteria for selecting this sample were far from reliable.

d) *Run-in phase*: Each study involved a run-in phase with the active drug before randomisation. While this creates the most favourable conditions for the drug to show its efficacy, it adversely affects external validity.

e) *Conflict of interest*: Both studies involved investigators with conflicts of interest relating to financial involvement with pharmaceutical companies. This, of course, is nothing unusual but it is of concern, especially given the changes to the protocol and the way in which the data were presented.

f) *Small treatment effects*: The treatment differences observed in EUROPA required large numbers of patients to achieve statistical significance – in fact, a composite primary end-point was needed to show an effect. Yet, there was no reduction in either cardiovascular or overall mortality. The PEACE study, on the other hand, showed no difference in the primary or secondary end-points.

g) *Assumption of the truth of* EUROPA: Interestingly, the response to the different findings between the two studies was to accept the truth of EUROPA and then try to account for the failure of PEACE to show the same effect. But why act as though PEACE is wrong? Why not assume EUROPA is wrong?

h) *Bias in the interpretation of data*: The authors of the PEACE study were unable to draw clear and unequivocal conclusions from their data. They appear to have expected the results to favour trandolapril and, no doubt, their sponsors were keen for the publication to do no harm to their product. The authors, it seems, fell into line by making excuses for the failure to show a benefit. Despite acknowledging that, in low-risk patients, there was no benefit from ACE inhibitors, this failed to prevent them from commenting that doctors may wish to consider using these drugs in patients who do not clearly fit the profile of patients in the study. Once again, the vested interest of the investigators is important.

i) *Latitude in the interpretation of data*: The controversy between EUROPA and PEACE emphasizes just how much leeway statistical studies leave to investigators in the interpretation of the results – so much so, that almost contradictory conclusions may be drawn from the same data.

j) *The failure of attempted replication*: The EUROPA and PEACE studies provide an excellent opportunity to show replication in action. Despite the arguments made by the authors of PEACE and various other commentators, the studies are very similar in terms of the design, the patients recruited and the treatment allocated. They each suffered from similar flaws including changes in protocol, the use of run-in phases and conflicts of interest. Furthermore – and most unusually – they were performed at very similar times. Despite this, conflicting results were obtained. But, instead of accepting the results and concluding that PEACE raised questions about the validity of EUROPA or vice versa, the differences in outcome were swept under the carpet. The clash between EUROPA and PEACE supports the contention that one RCT is unable to refute the findings of another.

Testing the Statistical Method

There's a distinction to be made between testing the result of an individual study and testing the statistical method in general. So far, we've considered whether or not the results of an individual RCT may be verified or falsified. The conclusion is that this isn't possible. It seems, then, that we simply have to take the results of any particular RCT on trust.

When it comes to testing the statistical method in general, the situation is even more difficult. As in the case of testing the results of a single large-scale RCT, individual instances or personal experience can play no role. We can't use epidemiological data to validate the statistical approach to research because it, too, uses a similar methodology. And, of course, it would be ridiculous to propose that RCTs might be used to validate their own methodology.

How, then, can we test the validity of the method used in statistics-based research? To do this, we would require something independent – something that doesn't involve statistics. Ideally, we would use the scientific method. But statistical studies were introduced precisely to deal with situations in which the standard method of investigating phenomena is unsuitable. Where the groups to be studied exhibit extreme heterogeneity – as in large-scale RCTs – the scientific method has no place. In such cases, there's no alternative to the statistical approach.

We have to recognise that there is no independent means of testing the validity of the methodology used in statistics-based research. There is, therefore, a dilemma: if we use statistical methods, we can't test their validity; if we don't use them, then we can't investigate some of the phenomena in the natural world. In other words, we have to choose between an unproven methodology and failing to investigate potentially important causal relationships. For those who are willing to put their faith blindly in statistical research, the course of action seems obvious. On the other hand, for those who demand evidence of the validity of the methodology, there's nothing lost by shunning statistics-based research because, whatever the outcome of these studies, we won't know whether anything of value has been found.

There is, though, a further point. If statistical studies were abandoned, researchers would have to turn their attention elsewhere. They'd be encouraged to spend more time and effort on basic science. They'd also be forced to seek out less and less heterogeneous groups. As the patients in RCTs become more homogeneous, the results would tend towards the scientific method. For example, there are many so-called risk factors – smoking, raised blood lipids, etc. – which, it's claimed, help to predict future cardiovascular events. Yet this information isn't used to deliver more homogeneous groups in RCTs. If we're really so accomplished at recognising risk factors, then surely we could create groups of patients with a very high risk – or, for that matter, with a genuinely very low risk?

Imagine the scenario where a group of patients has a 95% chance of a cardiovascular event over five years; and imagine that the drug reduces this to 50%. Now, there's a worthwhile result. But what about the losers? There would certainly be many. The whole of medical research would undergo upheaval. The professors would have to admit the error of their ways; so, too, would NICE and the Royal Colleges. Moreover, the approach to the management of millions of patients would be fundamentally changed. As for the pharmaceutical industry, their profits would be slashed. But, of course, these are simply the reasons why there will be no change.

Conclusions

When we hear a causal statement with which we are unfamiliar, we may doubt its truth. In which case, we ask for proof. This comes in the form of a demonstration. We expect that the relationship between a cause and its effect may be shown by an example. And what we see resolves our doubts. This is an integral part of causation.

Confirming and refuting the results of research is crucial to science and replication is the primary means by which this is achieved. But, as we've seen, there's no way of testing the results of any particular large-scale RCT or epidemiological study. Each study, as it were, is left hanging in the air, unsupported. Any doubts we may have about the validity of its results linger with little prospect of definitive confirmation or refutation.

Of greater importance, though, is the absence of means to test independently the validity of the method used in statistics based research. We can't use statistical studies without obvious circularity. As for the scientific method, it's clear that it has no role given the degree of heterogeneity to be found in the subject matter of statistical studies. The upshot of this, of course, is that we are effectively being asked to accept the methodology on the basis of trust.

References

1. Report of the Presidential Commission on the Space Shuttle Challenger Accident. June 6th 1986, Washington.
2. Penston J. *Fiction and Fantasy in Medical Research: the large-scale randomised trial.* The London Press. London, 2003.
3. Weiner MG, Xie D, Tannen RL. Replication of the Scandinavian Simvastatin Survival Study using a primary care medical record database prompted exploration of a new method to address unmeasured confounding. Pharmacoepidemiology and Drug Safety 2008;17;661-70.

4. Fox KM. Efficacy of perindopril in reduction of cardiovascular events among patients with stable coronary artery disease: randomised, double-blind, placebo-controlled, multicentre trial (the EUROPA study). Lancet 2003;362;782-88.
5. The PEACE investigators. Angiotensin-converting-enzyme inhibition in stable coronary artery disease. N Eng J Med 2004;351;2058-68.
6. Fox K, Ferrari R, Yusuf S, Borer JS. Should angiotensin-converting enzyme-inhibitors be used to improve outcome in patients with coronary artery disease and preserved left ventricular function? Eur Heart J 2006;27; 2154-7.

IX

A Reckless Act of Faith

If it's not possible to test the statistical method by any independent means, then we must either reject it or take it on trust. But to do so would be a reckless act of faith. We've already seen many instances of dubious practices relating to epidemiological studies and large-scale RCTs. In this chapter, we'll consider a prime example of all that is bad with modern-day medical research and one that should make us very wary of trusting those involved.

During the last few years, the Department of Health has introduced a national screening programme for colorectal cancer in England. What has occurred should rid us of any temptation to accept the claims of those who practice and use statistics-based research.

Colorectal Cancer Screening

The screening programme

Individuals aged 60-69 years of age receive a letter inviting them to participate in the NHS bowel cancer screening programme. Enclosed is a booklet – *Bowel Cancer Screening: The Facts*[1] – which purports to give the reader, "… information about bowel cancer, and the benefits and risks of bowel cancer screening." It explicitly claims to help individuals make an informed choice about participation. It tells them about the faecal occult blood test and discusses its accuracy. It warns of the risks of developing colorectal cancer. And it explains that the evidence shows that screening reduces the risk of dying from the disease by 16%.

About a week later, the test kit arrives. Two samples are taken from three consecutive bowel motions and returned by post. The faecal occult blood test demonstrates the presence of microscopic quantities of blood in the stool. If none of the samples contain blood, the test is negative; no further action is taken and the patient is invited for the second round of screening in two years time. If between one and four samples are positive, the result is classified as unclear and the test is repeated. If five or six samples are positive, the result is abnormal and the patient is advised to undergo colonoscopy.

The data

Evidence in favour of screening for colorectal cancer with faecal occult blood (FOB) testing comes from four large-scale RCTs carried out in the USA, Sweden, Denmark and the UK.[2-5] These studies were originally published in the 1990's but further papers on longer-term follow-up have subsequently appeared.[6-8]

RCTs of colorectal cancer screening using FOB testing

Location of study	Number of participants	Reduction in CRC mortality
USA	46,551	21%
Denmark	61,933	16%
Sweden	68,308	12%
UK	152,850	15%

The studies are similar in many respects. They all use the same faecal occult blood test although the processing varies with respect to the rehydration of samples which affects the sensitivity and specificity of the results. All used biennial testing but the US study also included an annual screening group. Sections of the populations, defined by age, were randomised to FOB testing or no intervention and followed up for long periods of time. The primary end-point in the four RCTs was mortality from colorectal cancer.

In 2008, an updated meta-analysis of the most recent data from the four RCTs was performed.[9] At first glance, the results look impressive. Pooling the studies produced data relating to more than 300,000 patients. The length of follow-up ranged between 11.7 and 18 years.

Including all participants, meta-analysis showed that screening with faecal occult blood tests reduced the mortality by 16%. When the analysis was restricted to biennial screening, the odds ratio was 0.85 (95% CI 0.78-0.92), giving a reduction in mortality of 15%. [9]

Meta-analysis of RCTs of Colorectal Cancer Screening (Biennial FOB Testing)

- 4 RCTs (Denmark, Sweden, USA, UK)
- Total participants 327,043

OR 0.85 (0.78-0.92)

15% reduction in mortality from colorectal cancer in the screening group compared with controls

This is the evidence on which the decision to introduce colorectal cancer screening with faecal occult blood tests in England was based. It is, however, nothing but a charade.

A failure of transparency about RCTs

Claims to provide sufficient information to enable the participants to make informed decisions don't hold water. No attempt has been made to explain the nature of the data from large-scale clinical trials.

As discussed earlier, a myth has been created that large-scale RCTs are the pinnacle of research. The opposite, however, the true: the larger the trial, the less reliable and the less worthwhile are the results. Even by the standards of recent times, the size of the RCTs in colorectal cancer screening is very large. The UK study, for example, involved more than 150,000 individuals. However, since the number of participants recruited is inversely proportional to the anticipated size of the effect, this should immediately raise suspicions about the value of any results. Not only are the advocates of screening silent about this matter, but they make every effort to hide the paltry size of the treatment effect.

There is also no mention of the many potential flaws in RCTs. For example, in relation to the studies of screening for colorectal cancer, the use of the double-blind technique was not an option.

Those invited to screening deserve to be informed about the fallibility of large-scale RCTs on which the programme is based and the failure of transparency in this regard is unacceptable.

The relative risk deception

As discussed in chapter V, researchers, sponsors and anyone who wishes to use the data from large-scale studies to promote a particular treatment usually present the results in terms of relative risk reductions. This is no accident. The use of relative risks creates the impression of a substantial treatment effect where actually none exists. It's nothing but a sleight of hand. Nowhere is this more obvious than in the case of colorectal cancer screening.

The information booklet accompanying the initial invitation to participate in screening claims that the process reduces mortality by 16%. This is repeated in the information sent to general practitioners. The data, in fact, show a reduction of 15% when the meta-analysis is confined to biennial screening, as used in the UK programme, but this distinction is conveniently ignored in the booklet. This, however, is a minor misdemeanour compared with the relative risk deception.

Let's accept, for a moment, that the relative risk reduction in mortality from colorectal cancer of 16% is an accurate estimate. Although it's tempting to believe that this applies to all individuals undergoing screening, this is far from the truth. It applies only to that small subgroup of individuals who would have died from colorectal cancer without screening.

Consider the results of the UK study of colorectal cancer screening.[5,7] During ten years of follow-up, less than 1% of controls died from colorectal cancer. The 16% reduction applies only to this tiny subgroup. For anyone considering participation in screening, the chances of benefit are remote. Firstly, they have be members of a subgroup comprising less than 1% of the population invited for screening who would die from colorectal cancer; secondly, they have to be in that minority of 16% of this very small subgroup in whom death would be prevented by screening. This is never explained in the information booklet.

Despite repeated criticisms of the use of relative risk reductions, data continue to be presented in these terms. The correct approach, however, is to present the results in the most straightforward way, that is, as absolute risk reductions. In UK study,[5,7] the absolute risk of dying from colorectal cancer in the controls was 0.8% over a period of ten years and this was reduced to 0.7% in those allocated to the screening group. Thus, the true reduction in mortality from colorectal cancer achieved by screening with faecal occult blood testing was 0.1% over ten years.

UK Study of Colorectal Cancer Screening

	Mortality from CRC over 10 years
Controls	0.8%
Screening	0.7%
Absolute risk reduction = 0.1%	
Death from colorectal cancer is prevented by screening in about 1/1000 individuals	

These data are to be found in the results section of the published papers. They do not, however, feature in the abstracts or in the discussion section. Reference is seldom made to the absolute risk reduction in presentations of colorectal cancer screening and certainly there is no evidence that patients are ever informed about the true size of the benefit.

The disease-specific mortality deception

The end-point of the RCTs of colorectal cancer screening is the mortality from colorectal cancer. But what if screening causes harm that leads to death in some patients? We have seen just how small the reduction in colorectal mortality is in the screened groups. Imagine if the screening process – which includes colonoscopy – causes just as many deaths as it prevents. In that case, the overall mortality would be the same in the screening group and controls. Indeed, re-analysis of the data from the RCTs has been reported as showing an increase in non-colorectal cancer deaths in the screening group compared with that in controls which balances the reduction in deaths from colorectal cancer attributed to screening.[10]

The overall death rate regardless of the cause – known as the all-cause mortality – is a better measure of the effect of screening than the disease-specific mortality used in the RCTs. It takes into account any unsuspected deaths resulting from the screening process.

As the meta-analysis makes clear,[9] there's no difference whatsoever between the all-cause mortality in the screening group and that in controls. It's not that there's a difference but that it isn't significant; the mortality is the same in the screened subjects and the controls. There is no "trend" suggesting a possible but unproven reduction in overall deaths in screened participants. The evidence is clear: the survival in those who participate isn't affected by screening.

All-cause Mortality in RCTs of Colorectal Cancer Screening with Faecal Occult Blood Testing (Meta-analysis)

OR = 1.0 (0.99-1.02)

No difference in overall mortality between the screening group and controls

Proponents of colorectal cancer screening argue that the reduction in mortality from colorectal cancer screening is lost in the all-cause mortality because the disease contributes only a small amount to the overall number of deaths. They also claim that to detect the small decrease in overall mortality would require RCTs involving millions of participants that would be very expensive and would take decades to complete. But these arguments rest on the assumption that the reduction in mortality due to screening reported in RCTs is a reliable finding and, more importantly, that screening doesn't cause deaths. Neither of these assumptions is acceptable.

CRC screening is being sold to the general public on the grounds that it saves lives. But there's no evidence for this claim. Those invited to screening aren't informed of the failure of RCTs to show any reduction in overall mortality. Yet the evidence is overwhelming. None of the four very large RCTs has demonstrated any reduction in all-cause mortality from screening. Moreover, pooling the data from more than 300,000 participants in a meta-analysis shows conclusively that there's no difference in survival between those who undergo screening and controls. This, of course, is seldom mentioned in discussions of colorectal cancer screening and, more importantly, is absent from the information booklets. It's nothing but a further deception.

The dangers of screening

Colonoscopy

As far as the information provided to participants is concerned, the only disadvantages of colorectal cancer screening relate to the procedure of colonoscopy.[1,11] The booklets do describe the risks of complications including perforation, haemorrhage and cardio-respiratory problems. However, whether they provide sufficient information for participants to appreciate fully the frequency and severity of these complications is open to debate and they certainly appear to minimize the risk of the procedure. For example, a large survey of colonoscopy performed in the UK and published in 2004 reported a risk of perforation of approximately 1/700, roughly twice that provided in the information booklets for colorectal cancer screening.[12]

Interestingly, nothing is said about the dangers of the bowel preparation. These include gastrointestinal side-effects – vomiting and abdominal pain – aspiration pneumonia, cardiac arrhythmias and a variety of metabolic disturbances such as hyperphosphataemia, hyponatraemia and hypokalaemia.[13] There are many reports in the literature of hyponatraemia caused by bowel preparation for colonoscopy [13-19] and this may lead to serious neurological damage and even death.[16-19]

Colonoscopy is not to be undertaken lightly. Most gastroenterologists will have personal experience of patients who developed serious complications or who died as a result of the procedure. This isn't reflected in the information given to patients nor in the way they are assessed before colonoscopy – this is left to nurses who lack the skills required to detect and interpret relevant clinical findings.

Psychological consequences of screening

Screening in general is associated with harm.[20] However, whilst the physical problems are obvious, psychological harm is often more subtle and is frequently neglected. We must remember that participation in screening disrupts the lives of otherwise healthy individuals. Many experience psychological stress.[21-26] This increases when they are informed that the initial test result is positive and continues even if later they are told that the result was a false positive.[21,27-32] Screening produces a state of increased awareness of illness [33-36] and some participants develop cancer phobias.[23,24] Finally, the risk of suicide is increased amongst patients with cancer [37-39] and it would seem prudent to avoid subjecting individuals with underlying psychological problems to the stress and worry of screening. Despite these findings, no mention is made of the psychological effects of screening in the information given to patients.

Colorectal cancer screening – as in the case of most screening programmes – isn't a benign process. It causes both physical and psychological harm. This is all the more reason why the benefits must be clearly and unequivocally demonstrated.

Breast Cancer Screening

There can be no excuses for the colorectal cancer screening programme. It's all happened before. Nobody, though, seems to have learned the lessons.

More than twenty years ago, breast cancer screening was introduced into the United Kingdom. What emerged in the ensuing years should have served as a warning to those wishing to embark on further screening programmes. As far back as 2001, some of the RCTs of breast cancer screening were criticised as being flawed and it was argued that using breast cancer mortality as the primary endpoint was misleading and biased in favour of screening.[40]

Michael Baum, a respected breast cancer surgeon who had been involved in screening from its inception, also raised concerns.[41]

> "I soon learned first hand the 'toxic side effects' of the process and became increasingly disturbed by the failure of true informed consent among innocent women who accepted the summons to the screening centre... It did not take me long to work out that the 25% relative risk reduction in breast cancer mortality headlined in the invitation could be framed in another way that described the absolute benefits..." [41]

As in the case of colorectal cancer, the results of RCTs were presented in terms of relative risk reductions which disguised the very small benefits of breast cancer screening.

A recent meta-analysis of the data further threatens the grounds for breast cancer screening.[42] Eight eligible trials involving 600,000 women were identified. One trial was excluded because of bias. The pooled data of four RCTs showed a reduction in breast cancer mortality attributed to screening of 25% but these studies had inadequate randomisation. When the analysis was restricted to the three RCTs with satisfactory randomisation, no reduction in breast cancer mortality was observed. More importantly, no difference in all-cause mortality was detected between the screening group and controls. The conclusion of the meta-analysis was that, for every 2000 women screened, one will avoid dying from breast cancer and ten healthy women – who would not have developed clinical breast cancer in their lifetime – will be treated unnecessarily with surgery, radiotherapy or chemotherapy; a further 200 will suffer from psychological distress as a result of false positive tests.[42]

Early in 2009, Gotzsche *et al.* published an article in the British Medical Journal in which they reiterated the findings of the meta-analysis.[43] They drew attention to the way in which benefits were exaggerated and harms minimised in information leaflets for breast cancer screening in the six countries studied. There was, for example, no mention of the serious problem of over-diagnosis, the false positive rates provided applied only to a single round of screening, and it was wrongly claimed that screening led to a reduction in surgery.

> "We believe that if policy makers had had the knowledge we now have when they decided to introduce screening 20 years ago, when nobody had published data on overdiagnosis or on the imbalance between numbers of prevented deaths and numbers of false positive screening results and the psychological consequences of the false alarms, we probably would not have had mammography screening."[43]

The article prompted a letter to *The Times* that was strongly critical of breast cancer screening.[44]

> "The most disturbing statistic is that none of the invitations for screening comes close to telling the truth. As a result, women are being manipulated, albeit unintentionally, into screening."[44]

We may take issue with the somewhat charitable interpretation that the data manipulation was unintentional. Those involved in the NHS breast cancer screening programme are intelligent, well-informed professionals who understand the nature of the data. Whilst it's possible that one or two individuals might make mistakes, it's inconceivable that the data manipulation and omissions wouldn't have been detected by others. It follows, therefore, that the very misleading presentation of breast cancer screening data was likely to have been intentional with the aim of promoting participation in the screening programme.

The Lessons from Cancer Screening

Screening for colorectal cancer epitomises statistics-based research in action. In earlier chapters, we've repeatedly seen how increasing the size of epidemiological studies and RCTs does nothing to improve the quality of the evidence gathered in support of causal relationships. The colorectal screening studies merely confirm this conclusion. Disputes about the validity of the data relating to cancer screening have been rife for a decade or more – again reflecting the uncertainties surrounding large-scale RCTs – while the problems with published studies that surface over time reinforce the many potential flaws with the statistical approach to research.

The invitation to the colorectal cancer screening programme gives the impression of providing sufficient and reliable evidence to enable individuals to make an informed decision about participation. But, in reality, it does nothing of the sort. The dangers of colonoscopy are underplayed and the psychological effects of the screening process are ignored. Nothing is said that might deter those invited to screening from participating. There isn't a word about the uncertainties of statistics-based research and nothing is said about the reason for performing large-scale RCTs – in other words, the very small treatment effects anticipated before the studies commence. Everything is done to hide the true size of the benefits. The use of the relative risk reduction and the lack of an explanation of what is involved in this measure, together with the failure to disclose the absolute risk reduction, are straightforward acts of deception. So, too, is the silence about the results of all four RCTs which demonstrate an absence of any reduction in all-cause mortality. There is no evidence that colorectal cancer screening increases survival.

The screening programme for colorectal cancer involves thousands of skilled and knowledgeable professionals from a variety of different disciplines – the researchers and academics who design and perform the studies, civil servants in the Department of Health, and NHS managers, not to mention the doctors and nurses who deliver the service. Yet, somehow, this army of professionals has delivered a screening service with no proven value. As judged by its uptake, the programme appears to be a success but this has only been achieved by widespread deception. Participants have been misled. So, too, have the general public who have to pay the enormous costs of the programme. But this isn't the first time. Similar acts of deception have persuaded millions of women to undergo screening for breast cancer. The scandal is that the whole process has been repeated.

But the focus on colorectal cancer screening serves another purpose. It provides a powerful argument against any suggestion that we should take the statistical approach to research simply on trust. The screening programme exposes data manipulation and deception on a grand scale. If the advocates of statistics-based research – whether those who design and perform the studies, or those who use the data – have no scruples about behaving dishonestly with the general public, their assurance that the methodology is sound is worthless.

References

1. Bowel cancer screening: the facts. NHS National Cancer Screening Programmes. Department of Health, UK.
2. Mandel JS, Bond JH, Church TR, et al. Reducing mortality form colorectal cancer by screening for fecal occult blood. N Eng J Med 1993;328; 1365-71.
3. Kewenter J, Brevinge H, Engaras B, et al. Results of screening, re-screening and follow-up in a prospective, randomised study for the detection of

colorectal cancer by fecal occult blood testing. Scand J Gastroenterol 1994;29;468-73.

4. Kronborg O, Fenger C, Olsen J, et al. Randomised study of screening for colorectal cancer with fecal occult blood test. Lancet 1996;348;1467-71.
5. Hardcastle JD, Chamberlain JO, Robinson MH, et al. Randomised controlled trial of faecal occult blood screening for colorectal cancer. Lancet 1996;348;1472-7.
6. Mandel JS, Church TR, Ederer F, et al. Colorectal cancer mortality: effectiveness of biennial screening for fecal occult blood. J Natl Cancer Inst 1999;91;434-7.
7. Scholefield JH, Moss S, Sufi F, et al. Effect of faecal occult blood screening on mortality from colorectal cancer: results from a randomised controlled trial. Gut 2002;50;840-4.
8. Kronborg O, Jorgensen OD, Fenger C, et al. Randomised study of biennial screening with a faecal occult blood test: results after nine screening rounds. Scand J Gastroenterol 2004;39;846-51.
9. Hewitson P, Glasziou P, Watson E, et al. Cochrane systematic review of colorectal cancer screening using the fecal occult blood test (Hemoccult): an update. Am J Gastroenterol 2008;103;1541-9.
10. Moayyedi P, Achkar E. Does fecal occult blood testing really reduce mortality? A reanalysis of systematic review data. Am J Gastroenterol 2006;101;380-4.
11. Bowel Cancer Screening: The Colonscopy Investigation. NHS Cancer Screening Programmes. Department of Health. 2006.
12. Bowles CJ, Leicester R, Romaya C, et al. A prospective study of colonoscopy practice in the UK today: are we adequately prepared for national colorectal cancer screening tomorrow? Gut 2004;53;277-83.
13. Wexner SD, Beck DE, Baron TH, et al. A consensus document on bowel preparation before colonoscopy. Gastrointest Endosc 2006;63;894-909.
14. Schroppel B, Segerer S, Kevneke C, et al. Hyponatraemic encephalopathy after preparation for colonoscopy. Gastrointest Endosc 2001;53;527-9.
15. Nagler J, Poppers D, Turetz M, et al. Severe hyponatraemia and seizure following a polyethylene glycol-based bowel preparation for colonoscopy. J Clin Gastroenterol 2006;40;558-9.

16. Dillon CE, Laher MS. The rapid development of hyponatraemia and seizures in an elderly patient following sodium picosulphate/magnesium citrate (Picolax). Age and ageing 2009;38;487.
17. Frizelle FA, Colls BM. Hyponatraemia and seizures after bowel preparation: report of three cases. Dis Colon Rectum 2004;48;393-6.
18. Ayus JC, Levine R, Arrieff AI. Fatal dysnatraemia caused by elective colonoscopy. Br J Med 2003;326;382-4.
19. Veitenhansl M, Reisch N, Schmauss S, et al. Hyponatraemic encephalopathy and rhabdomyolysis. Complications after preparation for colonoscopy with mannitol. Der Internist 2007;48;625-9.
20. Marshall KG. Prevention. How much harm? How much benefit? 3. Physical, psychological and social harm. Can Med Assoc J 1996;155;169-76.
21. Skrabanek P. False premises and false promises of breast cancer screening. Lancet 1985;2;316-20.
22. Stoate HG. Can health screening damage your health? J Roy Coll Gen Pract 1989;39;193-5.
23. Schmidt JG. The epidemiology of mass breast cancer screening – a plea for a valid measure of benefit. J Clin Epidemiol 1990;43;215-25.
24. Wardle J, Pope R. The psychological costs of screening for cancer. J Psychosomatic Res 1992;36;609-24.
25. Givens B, Oberle S, Lander J. Taking the jab out of needles. Can Nurse 1993;89;37-40.
26. Kottke TE, Trapp MA, Fores MM, et al. Cancer screening behaviors and attitudes in southeastern Minnesota. JAMA 1995;273;1099-1105.
27. Burton BK, Dillard RG, Clark EN. The psychological impact of false positive elevations of maternal serum α-foetoprotein. Am J Obstet Gynecol 1985;151;77-82.
28. Lerman C, Trock B, Rimer BK. Psychological and behavioural implications of abnormal mammograms. Ann Intern Med 1991;114;657-61.
29. Gram IT, Slenker SE. Cancer anxiety and attitudes toward mammography among screening attenders, non-attenders, and women never invited. Am J Public Health 1992;82;249-51.

30. Barton MB, Moore S, Polk S, Shtatland E, et al. Increased patient concern after false-positive mammograms: clinical documentation and subsequent ambulatory visits. J Gen Intern Med 2001;16;150-6.
31. Barton MB, Morley DS, Moore S, et al. Decreasing women's anxieties after abnormal mammograms: a controlled trial. J Natl Cancer Inst 2004;96; 529-38.
32. Brodersen J, Thorsen H, Kreiner S. Validation of a condition-specific measure for women having an abnormal screening mammography. Value in Health 2007;10;294-304.
33. White LS. The health care system. N Eng J Med 1975;293;773-4.
34. Thomas L. The healthy care system. N Eng J Med 1975;293;1245-6.
35. Fitzgerald FT. The qranny of health. N Eng J Med 1994;331;196-8.
36. Annas GJ. Reframing the debate on health care reform by replacing our metaphors. N Eng J Med 1995;332;744-7.
37. Fox BH, Stanek EJ, Boyd SC, et al. Suicide rates among cancer patients in Connecticut. J Chron Dis 1982;35;89-100.
38. Bolund C. Suicide and cancer: demographic and social characteristics of cancer. J Psychosoc Oncol 1985;3;17-30.
39. Kendal WS. Suicide and cancer. A gender comparison study. Ann Oncol 2007;18;381-7.
40. Gotzsche PC. Office of NHS cancer screening programme misrepresents Nordic work in breast screening row. BMJ 2001;323;1131 (letter).
41. Baum M. Ramifications of screening for breast cancer: Consent for screening. BMJ 2006;332;728.
42. Gotzsche PC, Nielsen M. Screening for breast cancer with mammography. Cochrane Database Syst Rev 2006;(4);CD001877.
43. Gotzsche PC, Hartling OJ, Nielsen M, et al. Breast screening: the facts – or maybe not. BMJ 2009;338;446-448.
44. Baum M, McCartney M, Thornton H, et al. Breast cancer screening peril: Negative consequences of the breast screening programme. *The Times*, 19th February 2009.

X

Hume *et al.*

Introduction

It's a common feature of research involving statistics that, in general, the studies are associated with very small differences in outcome between the groups. If the difference is found to be statistically significant, this is said to demonstrate the presence of a causal relationship. But is this inference justified?

The challenges to internal validity, the flaws in frequentist statistics and the possibility of fraud have already been discussed. These, together with the absence of any means of confirming the results of epidemiological studies and large-scale RCTs, give us every reason to doubt the validity of generalisations derived from statistics-based research.

But let's set aside these problems and assume that the conditions for internal validity have been fully satisfied and the frequentist theory is beyond reproach. Now, in these hypothetical circumstances, are we entitled to infer the presence of a causal relationship from a small, statistically significant difference? As soon as we ask this question, others surface. What is a causal relationship and how do we identify it? How does the particular type of causal relationship that emerges from statistical studies fit with that used in everyday life and science? Does statistics-based research deliver reliable causal generalisations? Are the predictions it supports reliable?

Here, we enter the realm of the philosophy of causation. This isn't a comfortable place. The subject is complex and the more we delve into it, the more difficulties we uncover. We soon find ourselves drowning in ever more obscure theories and suffocating in the never-ending counter examples to each of them. But, if we're to appreciate the problems with the statistical approach to causation, we have to grapple with the basic concepts.

There can be little debate about the starting point. Few would doubt the influence of David Hume's account of causation. Since the publication of *A Treatise of Human Nature* (1739)[1] and *An Enquiry into Human Understanding* (1748),[2] the regularity theory has dominated the subject. This isn't to say that it's remained unchallenged. On the contrary, it's become fashionable – amongst not only philosophers but also physicists and psychologists – to dismiss Hume's account. That there are flaws in the regularity theory is undeniable yet, of these, some are apparent, some are easily corrected while others are addressed by supplementing it with additional features. There are certainly inconsistencies in his texts and some of his ideas – especially in relation to his psychological account of causation – are frankly unsatisfactory. Moreover, there are differences between his earlier and later works reflecting the development of his thought. Nevertheless, as will be argued, Hume's insights remain of fundamental importance in understanding causation.

Theories of Causation

- Single case (direct perception) causation
- Regularity theory
- Necessary and sufficient conditions
- Counterfactual conditional theory
- Causation identified with fundamental properties of physics
- Causation and intervention
- Probabilistic (statistical) causation

In this chapter, the various accounts of causation will be discussed with particular emphasis on the regularity theory. However, probabilistic causation – which provides the basis for statistical research – will be addressed separately in the following chapter.

The Single Case – Are We Fooling Ourselves?

Hume begins his investigation with the observation of a single instance of causation. He draws attention to two obvious features of the relationship: a cause occurs before, and is proximal to, the effect.

> "Having thus discover'd or suppos'd the two relations of contiguity and succession to be essential to causes and effects, I find I am stopt short, and can proceed no farther in considering any single instance of cause and effect..." [3]

> "It appears that, in a single instance of the operation of bodies, we never can, by our utmost scrutiny, discover any thing but one event following another... All events seem entirely loose and separate. One event follows another; but we never can observe any tie between them. They seem conjoined, but never connected." [4]

The conclusion that we don't see anything other temporal priority and spatial contiguity in the single instance appears sound. Yet others don't view it this way. Many writers disagree with Hume and, instead, believe that we actually perceive causation when we observe a single instance of one event followed by another.[5-7] Ducasse, for example, asserted that, if we observe a situation in which A occurs immediately before and adjacent to B, and if A and B are the only changes occurring, then A is the cause of B.[5]

But how do we know that, in any particular instance, the two events that we observe are the only two that occur? How can we be sure that there isn't another factor – something that we fail to see – that causes the effect?

Ducasse contrives a situation in which we may be confident that there are only two events by limiting the field of observation to a tight space and time interface. But, even if we were to accept this, such circumstances are clearly not applicable to most cases in which we are considering a causal relationship. Where, for example, is the precise spatial and temporal interface between the cause and effect when, to use Fisher's example, fertilizer is added to the soil to increase the crop yield? Where is the interface between cause and effect when a drug is administered to abort a cardiac arrhythmia? How, exactly, is this to be directly observed?

More importantly, how do we know that the phenomenon will be repeated in the future? How can we be sure that our specification of the cause – its description, definition and measurement, etc. – is precise enough to allow us to reproduce the cause and effect relationship? We simply don't know that the phenomenon will be repeated. But, if we can't say that the inference from a single instance justifies a causal generalisation, then what use is it?

Causation and the Single Case

- There is nothing in a single instance of cause and effect other than spatial contiguity and temporal priority
- A single observation cannot provide evidence that the phenomenon will be repeated in future
- It has no application to most of scientific research
- Single case causation is convincing because we forget the background information involved in making these judgments

As Hume points out, when we appear to be drawing a causal inference from a single instance, we are, in fact, using previous experience and knowledge of similar phenomena.[8] We may be tempted to believe that we see causation in a single instance but this isn't the case. Were we able to rid ourselves of enough background knowledge, we would see the impossibility of making a reliable causal judgement based solely on the single instance.

Ducasse's theory and others like it have no relevance to most scientific research and, from the point of view of medical research, may be ignored. Those who support this view of causation need to specify what exactly it is – in addition to temporal priority and spatial contiguity – that they see when confronted with the single instance. Put another way, they must tell us what Hume neglected to see.

The Regularity Theory

Spatial contiguity and temporal priority are simply not sufficient. Something more is needed and Hume goes on to identify what he believes to be the primary feature of causation.

> "We remember to have had frequent instances of the existence of one species of objects; and also remember, that the individuals of another species of objects have always attended them, and have existed in a regular order of contiguity and succession with regard to them... Without any farther ceremony, we call the one cause and the other effect, and infer the existence of the one from that of the other" [9]

It's our repeated exposure to the constant relationship between two objects or events that leads us to infer the presence of a causal relationship.

> "The idea of cause and effect is deriv'd from experience, which informs us, that such particular objects, in all past instances, have been constantly conjoin'd with each other: And as an object similar to one of these is suppos'd to be immediately present in its impression, we thence presume on the existence of one similar to its usual attendant." [10]

These passages include two crucial components of the regularity theory: firstly, causal inference is derived from our experience of the natural world and, secondly, it's based on the presence of multiple observations involving two sets of similar objects or events related in terms of space and time. We make repeated observations of objects or events of type A; these are always followed closely in space and time by objects or events of type B; from this experience, we conclude that A causes B.

There are, of course, obvious problems with taking the regularity theory at face value. Opponents of Hume never cease to level the charge that correlation or concomitance is not causation. But he is fully aware of the dangers of accepting spurious causal relationships.

> "In almost all kinds of causes there is a complication of circumstances, of which some are essential, and others superfluous; some are absolutely requisite to the production of the effect, and others are only conjoin'd by accident." [11]

This quotation also shows that he is well acquainted with the complexity of nature and he takes great care when stepping into the minefield of causation. Indeed, he constructs a set of rules to assist in sifting out accidental or spurious associations from genuine causal relationships.

As we will see, the regularity theory is, by itself, insufficient to justify causal inference. Nonetheless, the feature of a regular association between cause and effect is crucial for reliable causal inference and for delivering universal causal generalisations.

The Regularity Theory of Causation

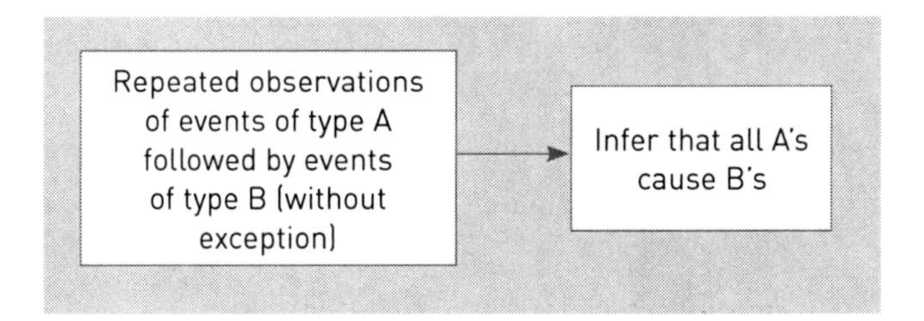

The Causal Connection

Hume's account describes what we actually do. But what grounds do we have for believing that it's legitimate to infer the presence of a causal relationship from repeated observations of A followed by B? As he points out, it's clear that the relationship between a cause and its effect can't be logical.

> "... there can be no demonstrative arguments to prove, that those instances, of which we have had no experience, resemble those of which we have had experience. We can at least conceive a change in the course of nature; which sufficiently proves, that such a change is not absolutely impossible. To form a clear idea of any thing, is an undeniable argument for its possibility, and is alone a refutation of any pretended demonstration against it. [12]

This argument rests on the idea that we can't imagine something illogical – for example, we can't imagine a four-sided triangle. Consider two propositions, "the cause occurs" (*p*) and "the effect occurs" (*q*). Now, let's assume that *p* logically entails *q*. If this is the case, the complex proposition [*p* and non-*q*] must be false – that is, the conjunction is logically impossible. Hence, we can't imagine it. Consequently, if we are able imagine a situation in which a cause isn't followed by the effect, the relationship between the two can't be logical.

The Causal Connection

- There is no necessary connection between a cause and its effect
- Causation involves distinct objects or events with no logical or analytic connection
- The causal relationship is contingent

Hume's argument is sound. Furthermore, as he observes, a cause and its effect are distinct events[13] and, as such, they can't be logically related to one another. Neither can the relationship be analytic – in other words, true by virtue of the meanings of the cause and its effect. Instead, our tendency to infer causation is grounded in the regularity which we observe.

> "For after a frequent repetition, I find, that upon the appearance of one of the objects, the mind is determin'd by custom to consider its usual attendant, and to consider it in a stronger light upon account of its relation to the first object. 'Tis this impression, then, or determination, which affords me the idea of necessity." [14]

We judge the presence of a causal relationship between A and B, at least in part, on the basis of our experience of their regular association. The grounds have nothing to do with links between the cause and its effect in terms of logic or meaning and there's no necessary connection. There are no necessary causes in nature.

Necessary and Sufficient Causes

Theories based on necessary and sufficient causes occur commonly in the philosophical literature.[15-17] In this context, the terms "necessary" and "sufficient" don't involve logical or analytic truths but are used in a weaker sense. When we use them, we must be careful to avoid implying anything other than that of relationships between events in the natural world.

When we say that C is a necessary cause of E, we mean nothing more than that, in the normal course of events, E wouldn't occur without C. The practical implication of this is that if C is prevented, then we can prevent E. Similarly, when we claim that C is a sufficient cause of E, this entails that if C occurs, then E would follow. According to this relationship, if we introduce C, we can reliably bring about the occurrence of E.

Theories of causation based on necessary and sufficient causes are generally believed to be inadequate. Many of the arguments used, though, are far from convincing.

There are no strictly necessary or sufficient causes

On a purely logical interpretation, it's always possible to argue that there are no strictly necessary or sufficient causes. There's no reason to believe that there's only one cause for a particular effect and, hence, no cause can be deemed necessary. Similarly, we don't have to accept that any particular cause will always be followed by its effect and, hence, no cause can be considered sufficient.

But, if we have grounds for believing that the background conditions are constant with respect to other relevant factors and if, under these circumstances, experiments have repeatedly shown that the effect doesn't occur in the absence of the cause, we may use this information to prevent the occurrence of the effect in future. Similarly, if experiments show that the cause is always followed by the effect, then we're able to produce the effect by introducing the cause under the same conditions. When interpreted in this weaker sense, the concepts of necessary and sufficient causes have practical value and a justified use.

Loss of asymmetry between cause and effect

Another criticism used against theories involving necessary and sufficient causes is that they destroy the asymmetry which is an integral part of causation – namely, if C causes E, E does not cause C.

In logical terms, if *p* is both necessary and sufficient for *q*, then *q* is both necessary and sufficient for *p*. Hence, if a cause is both necessary and sufficient for its effect, then the effect is necessary and sufficient for the cause. It follows that, if the identification of a causal relationship rests on the notions of necessary and sufficient causes, we can't tell the difference between cause and effect. But this is not how the words "necessary" and sufficient" are used in the context of causation. A cause and its effect are distinct, logically independent events. In any case, this problem is readily resolved by taking temporal priority and intervention into account, both of which distinguish a cause from its effect.

Compound causes

There are situations in which the ideas of necessary and sufficient causes appear to be unsuitable. Consider the case where two factors, C_1 and C_2, are both required for the occurrence of the effect, E. Alone, neither C_1 nor C_2 is followed by E. Here, C_1 and C_2 are compound causes and neither may be considered to be *the* cause. In such situations, we usually choose to make either C_1 or C_2 part of the background conditions leaving the other to be counted as the cause.

Causal over-determination

If C_1 and C_2 are each sufficient to produce E, then which ever occurs is the cause of E. But when both are present, this is said to bring into question the notion of causation based on necessary and sufficient conditions. The standard example is that of a firing squad where no individual member may be said to be a necessary cause of the death of the prisoner. The problem of multiple causes may often be resolved by closer inspection of the event in question. We may find, for example, that C_1 or C_2 occurred first, or there may be reason to believe that one or other produced the effect in the particular circumstances. Given additional information, we may be able to identify the precise cause.

However, when it comes to research, potential causes are identified and studied individually in experiments and randomised trials, thus excluding the problems of causal over-determination.

Dependence on regularity theory

The charges commonly levelled against the idea of necessary and sufficient causes turn out to be more apparent than real. The terms are often used in everyday life, as well as in science, without problems. They're useful shorthand expressions that summarise particular types of causal relationships. For example, when we speak of a necessary cause, we imply that, other things being equal, the effect wouldn't occur in the absence of the cause, and that removing the cause in future would prevent the occurrence of the effect. As Mackie showed,[17] the concepts may be applied to numerous individual situations as long as due consideration is given to the background circumstances.

However, when it comes to providing an account of causation, there is a more serious objection. If we claim that C is a necessary cause of E, then it follows that E doesn't occur in the absence of C. Similarly, if C is claimed to be a sufficient cause of E, then all instances of C are followed by E. But these statements can only be made if there's evidence in the form of consistent observations. In other words, theories based on necessary and sufficient causes depend on Hume's regularity theory. Thus, they cannot by themselves be said to provide a satisfactory account of causation.

The Origin of the Belief in Causation

As we've seen, Hume rejects the notion of a necessary connection between cause and effect. Our ideas of causation relate to distinct, logically independent events in the natural world and are the result of our experiences. He also dismisses the account, proposed by John Locke,[18] that causation is somehow related to a power which the cause has to produce its effect.[19-21] He argues strongly that postulating that a cause has a secret power doesn't achieve anything. We have no knowledge of such a power and we can't know that it would operate in future.

What, then, is the origin of our belief in causation? It's characteristic of Hume's philosophy that, whenever nature comes face to face with reason, nature triumphs. Whether it's in the context of our belief in the existence of external objects or the origin of morality, it's our nature which ultimately provides the explanation. And it's no different when it comes to drawing causal inferences.

Hume turns to psychology. If our previous experiences have always been of A followed by B, then the further occurrence of A produces the idea of B in our minds.[22-24] This is an automatic, immediate association of ideas. Thus, causal inference is grounded in psychological mechanisms – in our nature, not in our reason.

> "... we are determined by custom alone to expect the one from the appearance of the other. This hypothesis seems even the only one which explains the difficulty, why we draw from a thousand

> instances, an inference which we are not able to draw from one instance, that is, in no respect, different from them... All inferences from experience, therefore, are effects of custom, not of reasoning."[25]

Accordingly, causation is grounded in custom or habit. In most cases, causal inference involves no thought or consideration. It just happens. However in certain circumstances, we may use our intellect to reflect on matters and examine whether or not a causal relationship is present.[26]

Hume's psychological theory hasn't stood the test of time and justifiably has been the target of widespread criticism. Moreover, there is circularity in his arguments because his account assumes causation. The occurrence of A produces – or causes – the impression or idea of A in the mind which, in turn, produces – or causes – the idea of B. But, whilst the psychological aspects are undoubtedly flawed, this doesn't entail that his theory of causation is beyond redemption.

Bennett has proposed replacing Hume's "habit" or "custom" with dispositions.[27] This change involves speaking only of our disposition to expect B when we're presented A. In other words, we're to focus on what people actually do without reference to the possible cause of why they behave in the way they do. This leaves the fundamental features of Hume's theory intact while ridding it of the flawed psychological analysis and its inherent circularity.

As Bennett makes clear, this relatively small adjustment preserves much of Hume's regularity theory.[27] It allows the claim that causal relationships are based on the identification of regularity in repeated instances and that these may be generalised to future cases. The notion of causation remains grounded in our nature. We have certain dispositions and one of these is to interpret regularity and resemblance in terms of causation. When we act in line with this disposition, we are obeying a rule which states that when objects or events are related to one another in terms of space and time, and when this relationship is maintained throughout many observations, then we are to infer that the earlier event causes the later event. Thus, when these conditions are satisfied, we conclude that a causal relationship is present. This is simply what we do. It's in our nature. There's no further explanation.

This account may seem trivial. But, for Hume, nothing could be further from the truth. In the *Enquiry*, he emphasizes the importance of causation in the conduct of our daily lives.[28,29] It's essential for all our actions. Without it, we couldn't act with purpose, we couldn't change the world around us and, most importantly, we couldn't bring about outcomes that are beneficial or avoid those which are detrimental to us.

Because of its crucial role, we have to have a way of identifying cause and effect relationships that is subject to the least error.

> "...this operation of the mind, by which we infer like effects from like causes, and vice versa, is so essential to the substance of all human creatures, it is not probable, that is could be trusted to the fallacious deductions of our reason, which is... extremely liable to error and mistake. It is more conformable to the ordinary wisdom of nature to secure so necessary an act of the mind, by some instinct or mechanical tendency, which may be infallible in its operations... nature has implanted in us an instinct, which carries forward the thought in a correspondent course to that which she has established among external objects..." [29]

For Hume, causal inference is too important to be left to the frailties of our intellect. Instead, it's instinctive, automatic and reliable. This isn't to say that we can't ponder cause and effect relationships – clearly, we do so. We discuss causes and effects, and argue about the consequences of changes in the world around us. But, in many instances, we simply act in line with our disposition without giving it a second thought.

Psychology and Causation

An alternative approach to the investigations of causation is to be found in the field of psychology. Here, the method of philosophy is replaced by experiments which are believed to shed light on how we draw causal inferences.

According to psychologists, children as young as three months show behaviour suggestive of some understanding of causal phenomena. For example, infants are reported to be surprised when solid objects appear to break into fragments spontaneously, to pass through one another, to fail to exhibit a particular trajectory or to hang unsupported in the air without falling to the ground.[30,31] But is a three-month old child looking surprised really sufficient to infer that they have causal understanding? The problems of interpreting the results of such studies in infants are well recognised.

There's no doubt, however, that children learn causal concepts from an early age.[32] Schulz and Gopnik cite many studies that show that, by the age of four years, children are able to draw causal inferences related to simple ideas about physics, biology and psychology.[32] For example, they can understand causal relationships between the movement of objects, what makes organisms grow, and how human behaviour is affected by beliefs and emotions. In each of these areas, they make appropriate predictions, provide causal explanations and even use counterfactual conditionals.[32]

Psychologists are confident that they know a great deal about children's knowledge of causation at various ages but they admit that they know little about how children actually learn about the subject. This is not for want of trying – on the contrary, it's just that the experimental evidence is inconclusive.[32] Psychologists, for instance, can't agree on the primary means by which children learn about causal relationships.[33,34] In many ways, their disputes mirror those in philosophy. Some favour Ducasse's view of direct perception of causation in a single instance while others believe that children learn by observing regularity in line with Hume's theory. There as those who think that children identify causation by having pre-existing knowledge of causal mechanisms. And there are also those who prefer a less rigid approach and consider that different methods of learning are appropriate to different situations. Thus, there seem to be as many theories of how children might learn causation as there are about causation itself.

In adults, experiments in the psychology of causation produce equally unclear outcomes. We only have to consider the famous experiments performed by Michotte more than 60 years ago.[35] Observers watched a screen on which shape X moved towards shape Y. When X touched Y, X stopped and Y began to move in the same direction in which X had been moving. The process was repeated, varying both the ratio of the velocities of the two shapes (X/Y) and the interval between X coming to a halt and Y starting to move. Michotte found that if the velocity ratio was between five and ten, and the delay was <50msecs, observers stated that the movement of X caused the movement of Y. However, if the velocity ratio was <1, they failed to report the presence of a causal relationship. Causation was also said to be absent when a change in colour of X, instead of movement of X, was followed by movement in Y.

The results of the experiment led Michotte to conclude that the perception of causation couldn't be based on regularity and, hence, that Hume was wrong. In addition, since observers reported causation only under certain circumstances, he claimed that this reflected a direct observation of the particular features characteristic of causation. Human responses to experiences of single events, he asserted, are immediate and innate. In effect, he believed that his experiments showed that we actually perceive causation directly.

Michotte's work, however, has been criticised on many fronts, including his selection of subjects and the experimental methods used. Moreover, there have been difficulties in replicating his results. But even if the methodological issues were excluded, there remains a fundamental problem relating to the interpretation of the results. The conditions of the experiment were contrived and hardly reflect natural situations. Any reasonable observer – aware that the images on the screen were programmed events with no causal connection between the movements of the shapes – would have rejected any suggestion of a causal relationship. Causation is set in the real world, not on screens, and our causal judgments are made about actual events in the relevant context and set against a background of knowledge and experience.

Psychologists have been involved with the study of causation for many decades yet their contributions to the ontology and epistemology of this subject have been limited. This is only to be expected. The problems of causation are conceptual, not empirical and, hence, the experimental method is unlikely to shed light on the matter.

Hume's Definitions of Cause

In each of his two major works, Hume provides two definitions of a cause. Both pairs of definitions share features in common. In the *Treatise*, he describes the first definition of a cause as philosophical and the second as natural or psychological.

> "An object precedent and contiguous to another, and where all the objects resembling the former are plac'd in like relations of precedency and contiguity to those objects, that resemble the latter."[36]

> "... an object precedent and contiguous to another, and so united with it, that the idea of the one determines the mind to form the idea of the other, and the impression of the one to form a more lively idea of the other." [36]

In the *Enquiry*, while he keeps the classification in terms of philosophical and psychological definitions, there are obvious differences.

> "...an object, followed by another, and where all the objects similar to the first are followed by objects similar to the second. Or, in other words, where, if the first object had not been, the second had never existed." [37]

> "... an object followed by another, and whose appearance always conveys the thought to that other." [37]

The development in Hume's thinking is readily apparent. The later philosophical definition dispenses with the requirement for contiguity, perhaps because of his increasing awareness of scientific discoveries showing how objects may act on each other over vast distances, as in the case of gravity. Furthermore, almost as an aside, the philosophical definition in the *Enquiry* includes a counterfactual conditional statement which was absent from the earlier version.

In Hume's account, the philosophical definitions stipulate the conditions for the establishment of a causal relationship whereas the psychological definitions show how causation is grounded in our nature.

Counterfactual Theory of Causation

At first glance, Hume's addition of the counterfactual conditional to his definition of causation in the *Enquiry* appears so innocent. We feel comfortable with counterfactuals in this context and we use them, often in an informal style, to express a particular feature of causal relationships. Some philosophers, however, have interpreted Hume's remark differently; for them, the counterfactual conditional is the essence of causation.

David Lewis, one of the most influential writers on the subject, welcomes Hume's "other words" and interprets them as the basis for an entirely new approach to causation.[38]

> "... we do know that causation has something or other to do with counterfactuals. We think of a cause as something that makes a difference, and the difference it makes must be a difference from what would have happened without it. Had it been absent, its effects – some of them, at least, and usually all – would have been absent as well." [38]

The counterfactual theory is applied to individual instances of causation. Event *c* occurs and causes event *e*. Whether or not this is a genuine case of causation depends on the truth of the counterfactual conditional statement that if *c* hadn't occurred, then *e* wouldn't have occurred. On this view, it's the presence of a counterfactual relationship between two events that establishes causation.

The need for possible worlds

Immediately, though, there's a problem. As Lewis remarks, counterfactual conditionals are poorly understood, especially when subjected to analysis. We know that event *c* did not occur and, therefore, that the antecedent of the counterfactual is false. This presents difficulties for standard propositional logic. If the antecedent is false, the counterfactual conditional is true regardless of the truth of the consequent. Thus, simply by ensuring that the antecedent is false, we would guarantee the truth of any counterfactual conditional and, as a consequence, its truth would be trivial.

Lewis's solution is to introduce the notion of possible worlds. The truth-conditions of counterfactuals are presented in terms of the relationships between possible worlds. The counterfactual "if *c* hadn't occurred, then *e* wouldn't have occurred" is true if and only if there is a possible world in which both the antecedent and the consequent are true that is closer to the actual world than any other possible world in which the antecedent is true and the consequent is false. Although false in the real world, the antecedent may be considered true in other possible worlds that have a different history from our world. But, the introduction of possible worlds is not to everyone's liking.

Other challenges to the counterfactual theory

Talk of possible worlds is only the start of the journey to cope with all of the demands raised by Lewis's theory of causation.

The counterfactual relationship fails to provide the necessary asymmetry that allows for the identification of the direction of causation. The usual approach – and the one favoured by Hume – is to use temporal priority in order to distinguish cause from effect. This solution, however, is rejected by many philosophers on the grounds that it precludes both backwards causation and the use of causation to explain the direction of time, and that there are practical problems involved in the timing when events occur simultaneously.

Then there is the problem of epiphenomena. Consider the case where C first causes X and then causes E, although X doesn't cause E. Suppose also that C always causes E and that E is only caused by C – in other words, C is a necessary and sufficient cause of E. In this situation, X is said to be an epiphenomenon. But, if X hadn't occurred, E wouldn't have occurred and so, if we adopt the counterfactual approach to causation, this supports the claim that X causes E which is, of course, spurious.

A further problem for the counterfactual analysis is causal pre-emption. Consider the situation where C_1 and C_2 each cause E. Both occur but, in this particular case, only C_1 causes E. Had C_1 not occurred, C_2 would have caused E. Thus, C_2 is a potential cause of E but is pre-empted by C_1. This is a case of over-determination and it results in flawed counterfactual analysis. If C_1 hadn't occurred, it's not the case that E wouldn't have occurred because it would still have been brought about by C_2.

The presence of a counterfactual relationship isn't sufficient for the establishment of causation. The dependency expressed by counterfactual conditionals is considerably broader than that of causal dependency. Consider, for example, the statement, "If yesterday hadn't been Christmas Day, then today wouldn't be Boxing Day." This is a counterfactual conditional but the relationship to which it refers isn't causal but analytic – in other words, it's true by virtue of the meanings of the terms "Christmas Day" and "Boxing Day". Causal dependence is just one of a number of dependency relationships that can be expressed by counterfactuals.[39]

In order to defend the counterfactual theory of causation, Lewis proposes solutions that, although novel and clever, are too far-fetched for many palates. Indeed, many find his account unconvincing.[40]

What does it all mean?

For the past forty years, counterfactual analysis has provided a rich vein of ideas to be mined by philosophers. But, when it comes to an account of causation, the product of all this industry is unimpressive. As challenges to the validity of the theory emerge, the proponents of counterfactual analysis patch up the damage but the repairs are themselves the source of even greater dissatisfaction.

> "However, one cannot help but have the sinking feeling that we are heading for an interminable series of objections and modifications, and that even if there is an end result, it will not have the simplicity and intuitive appeal that recommended the original version." [40]

The problems, however, were there right at the start. As Lewis correctly pointed out in 1973, counterfactuals are "ill understood".[38] But further analysis hasn't really helped – it's just made matters worse. If we are to understand these odd parts of our language, we should look more closely at how we actually use them.

Consider a previously healthy young adult who is given insulin in error resulting in death. The counterfactual statement, "If the John Smith hadn't been given the insulin, then he wouldn't have died," could be used in many different situations. It may be uttered by the doctor who prescribed the drug as an admission of responsibility or by the nurse who failed to notice the mistake in order to express her regret. It may be used by angry relatives to point the finger of blame at those involved. Or it may be a warning from those campaigning against medical errors.

These uses of the counterfactual conditionals have reference to causation. But what exactly is the link? We have to consider the context. We know what actually occurred: the man was given insulin by mistake and subsequently died. From this event, we draw a causal inference. This is based on our knowledge of actions of insulin – that it causes hypoglycaemia which, in turn, disturbs cerebral function leading to brain damage and death. Our knowledge of these causal relationships is grounded in the regularity theory. Depending on the dose, insulin always causes hypoglycaemia. The evidence for this generalisation is extensive and consistent. It's against this background that we use the counterfactual conditional, "If John Smith hadn't been given the overdose of insulin, then he wouldn't have died." On the other hand, if his death been preceded closely in time by a pin being stuck into an effigy of him, we wouldn't say, "If the pin hadn't been stuck into the effigy, then John Smith wouldn't have died," because we don't – or most of us don't – believe in Voodoo. In this case, the background circumstances used to justify the use of a counterfactual conditional are lacking.

It's not that the counterfactual conditional relationship establishes causation. On the contrary, we are justified in using a counterfactual conditional statement because causation has already been established.

The counterfactual conditional is a type of expression that we use in relation to causal situations that serves certain purposes. It's based on much information relevant to the particular causal context and, as such, may be considered to be shorthand for the totality of grounds on which the counterfactual is based. In this sense, it resembles Mackie's view of counterfactuals as being condensed arguments.[41]

The Counterfactual Theory of Causation

- Applies to single cases of causation
- Relies on the theory of possible worlds
- Fails to account for causal asymmetry
- Challenged by epiphenomena and causal pre-emption
- Counterfactual relationship is too broad
- Dependent upon background causal knowledge derived from regularity theory

As noted above, the counterfactual analysis is applied to individual cases of causation. Without any reference to other knowledge, causal inference would be impossible unless we were to accept that we are able to observe causation directly. But this approach to causation is unsatisfactory.

Counterfactual conditionals are dependent on previously established causal relationships and, thus, can't be used to identify causation. They are a turn of phrase, a way of speaking that encapsulates one aspect of the causal relationship. Interpreted in this way, Hume's "other words" make sense.

Causation and Science

Hume, no doubt, would be dismissive of the claims of modern-day physicists and philosophers to have hit upon the true nature of causation.

> "... the ultimate force and efficacy of nature is perfectly unknown to us; and that 'tis in vain we search for it in the known qualities of matter." [42]

In recent decades, there's been increasing interest in scientific explanations of causation and, in particular, the identification of causation with the transfer of energy or momentum.

Salmon introduced the idea of a causal process.[43] This is the means by which causal influence is propagated from one location to another. He gives the following example. A ball is hit by a bat; this is an event, or causal interaction, and is short-lived. The ball then travels through the air; this is a causal process with longer duration. Then the ball strikes the window and breaks the glass; again, this is a causal interaction. In this case, the causal process has transmitted energy from the first to the second event. Thus, when events or interactions occur, energy and momentum are transferred.

The identification of causation with fundamental physical processes may be of interest to scientists. But how relevant is this approach? It's strictly applicable only to a few instances of causation. In particular, it depends on structures and events at a micro level and, as such, has little relevance to most situations. Physicists may choose to explain causation in terms of energy transfer but how is such an approach to be accommodated in other areas? What are researchers in biology, psychology or the social sciences to make of it? Where does energy transfer at a micro level fit in with epidemiological studies or randomised trials in medical research?

Causal concepts are part of our everyday language and there's little in the way we normally speak of one event causing another that bears any resemblance to ideas of the transfer of energy or momentum.

In contrast to the enthusiasm of modern day physicists and philosophers, Hume was sanguine about the chances of identifying the true nature of the causal connection.

> "... philosophers who carry their scrutiny a little farther, immediately perceive that, even in the most familiar events, the energy of the cause is as unintelligible as in the most unusual, and that we only learn by experience the frequent conjunction of objects, without being ever able to comprehend anything like connexion between them." [44]

In Salmon's example of the ball breaking the window, the energy of the ball is said to be transferred to the glass. But, in Hume's terms, what we observe is a ball moving through the air and hitting the window followed by the breaking of the glass. As we delve into the problem more deeply, we may think that we will eventually encounter the essence of causation. But is this really so? And why should we stop there?

> "The most perfect philosophy of the natural kind only staves off our ignorance a little longer." [45]

Interesting though the scientific account of causation is, it has little to do with what we normally consider to be cause and effect relationships. And it certainly has no place in most statistics-based research.

The Role of Intervention in Determining Causation

Perhaps we should begin with some of the commonly used arguments against including deliberate intervention in any theory of causation. Philosophers, it appears, aren't keen on the idea of giving human action a role. Mackie referred to the "*... deplorable anthropocentricity of talk of interventions.*" [17] There's dissatisfaction, too, with the way any theory based on intervention fails to offer a comprehensive account. It precludes causation involving the more remote parts of space and time. For example, intervention isn't possible in geology where events occurred many millions of years ago and we aren't able to manipulate the movements of the planets or stars to determine the outcome of our actions. But, perhaps the most serious problem is that causation is viewed as the more basic idea and, so the argument goes, it can't be grounded on intervention.

These criticisms, however, are not insurmountable. We could restrict our consideration of causation to those parts of space and time that are accessible to intervention. Excluding the inaccessible regions would have little impact on the vast majority of occasions on which we investigate causation. As for the other criticisms, they are primarily concerned with the ontology of causation – in other words, with what it means for an object or event to be a cause. But we may easily set such questions aside and focus instead on the epistemology of causation. This may not be welcomed by philosophers. But the rewards surely outweigh their qualms.

Hume's implicit intervention

The notion of intervening in the course of events in the natural world is integral to causation. The primary purpose of identifying causal relationships is to enable us to change outcomes so as to promote those we desire and to prevent those we wish to avoid. As Hume notes, without causation…

> "We should never know how to adjust means to ends, or to employ our natural powers in the production of any effect. There would be an end at once of all action, as well as of the chief part of speculation." [28]

Clearly, he links causation with intervention but this doesn't form part of his account of causation. Indeed, most of his remarks appear to refer to observational instances. The examples he gives, however, suggest that intervention is bound up with causation.[46-48] He speaks of the interaction between billiard balls, of the effect of on objects left unsupported above the ground, of fire burning and water suffocating humans. He comments on how causation is involved in the growth of plants, the reproduction in animals, and the nourishment of bodies by food. And, he discusses the purgative effects of rhubarb and the soporific action of opium.

When we consider both Hume's view of the practical importance of causation in our lives and the examples which he chooses, it's not hard to conclude that he must realise the central role of intervention in the identification of causal relationships. He is certainly acquainted with experimental science and the role of manipulating the conditions in order to identify causal relationships.[49]

Hume, it seems, takes intervention for granted and simply expects us to recognise its essential role in causation without any further comment. When it comes to the deliberate manipulation of a cause with the intention of observing the occurrence of the effect, he is silent. He may believe that intervention is a fundamental feature of causation but everything is implicit.

Von Wright's account of causation

GH von Wright, on the other hand, gives an account of causation in which intervention explicitly plays a central role.[50] It is epistemological rather than ontological – it deals with how we come to identify causal relationships instead of focusing on the nature of causation.

The account is based on the regularity theory.[50] This is essential in order to provide a stable background against which to judge the effect of intervention. If we observe both the regular occurrence of the C followed the E and the non-occurrence of E when C is absent, we have stable background conditions. But, by themselves, these observations aren't enough to justify causal inference. They fail to exclude either that C and E are only accidentally associated or that they are each the effect of a common cause.

According to von Wright,[50] intervention involves a change in the course of nature – something occurs which, without the intervention, would not have occurred. Thus, he includes elements of the counterfactual theory in his account. But we have to be sure that the outcome would not have occurred in the absence of the intervention. This is the requirement for regularity. Necessary and sufficient conditions are supported by the regularity theory and protected by intervention from the common challenges levelled against them.

But that's not all. Intervention establishes the direction of causation by distinguishing the cause from the effect. Manipulating C produces E but manipulating E doesn't produce C; hence, the direction of causation becomes clear. This is of particular relevance in the context of functional laws. In the case of the gas laws, for example, changes in temperature are associated with changes in pressure. But which is the cause and which is the effect? Intervention solves this problem. If we manipulate the temperature and observe a change in pressure, then – in these circumstances – it's the change in temperature that causes the change in pressure. Without intervention, it isn't possible to speak of causation in this setting.

The observation of the regular association between C and E becomes a causal relationship when it is confirmed by experiment. This is how causation is established and it leads to causal laws.

Needless to say, von Wright's theory has been heavily criticised for reasons discussed above. But his emphasis on epistemology – that is, describing the conditions under which we may reliably identify causal relationships – goes some way to deflecting many of the criticisms while the central role of intervention brings causation into the practical sphere where it belongs.

Causation – regularity theory plus intervention

In many ways, supplementing Hume's regularity theory with intervention provides a satisfactory account of how we identify causal relationships.

In science, for example, the slogan "regularity plus intervention" would describe the means by which causal relationships are identified. We use controls to show what occurs when the cause is missing and we compare this outcome with that observed when the intervention is present. The strength of the scientific method resides in our ability to identify homogeneous classes of objects with respect of the outcome. Given standard conditions, pure water freezes at 0°C; this is constant and predictable; every time we repeat this observation, the result is the same. Similarly, the addition of sodium chloride prevents water freezing at 0°C; again, this is entirely predictable; each time the intervention is present, the outcome is the same. And, of course, intervention allows us to be sure that the only change in the conditions is the addition of salt. Reliable causal inference is grounded in the regularity observed in each of the groups studied and in the act of intervention which guarantees the isolation of the single factor involved in the production of the effect.

As Hume made clear, causation is of the utmost importance. But its importance doesn't lie in philosophical theories. It's a practical matter. We act in a certain way and this yields results. The scientific method is merely a formal approach to what we do naturally in the course of our lives. What we're really interested in is the practical consequences of behaving in a particular way. We want to be able to manipulate the natural world to our advantage. We want a reliable way to make changes, something that's going to yield predictable outcomes. And the best way to do this is to use the regularity theory allied to intervention. If we want to identify a cause – something that brings about a change – what better way than to use deliberate intervention to promote or prevent its effect.

Everyday Notions of Causation

If the regularity theory bolstered by intervention is the preferred candidate for an account of causation, then we should expect to find evidence for this in our words and actions in everyday situations. Our language should reflect those features of causal relationships which are consistent with such a theory.

Learning about causation

The early years

Imagine watching an infant in her cot. She picks up the rattle and shakes it. It makes a noise. She repeats the action, again and again, each time with the same result. Sitting in her high chair, she sees that the bowl containing her food always moves when she pushes it and the plastic cup always falls to the floor when she lets go. Every morning, she watches her mother pull back the curtains to fill the room with sunlight and every evening a flick of the light switch sends the bedroom into darkness. The world around the infant is full of causal regularities. What's more, there's a regular link between her actions and the outcomes. This offers a background, a framework, against which causal language is learned.

Consider the pop-up toys popular amongst toddlers. A row of closed boxes are individually opened by pressing a button at the base of each box. From each opened box springs up a different animal. We teach the child to play – showing her how to press the buttons to open the boxes and pointing to the different animals appearing from each box. We coax her to bring up a specific animal. "Where's the rabbit?" And if she stumbles, we take over. "No, the rabbit's in this box. Push this button. Look, there's the rabbit." She soon learns which box contains each animal and how to bring up the rabbit. But what if pressing one particular button opened the boxes at random? What if pressing the button often had no effect? What if the animals somehow changed position whilst the boxes were closed? Worse, what if all of these conditions were present? It may be entertaining, but without the regularity, she couldn't learn anything about making a particular animal appear. In fact, she couldn't even be sure that anything would happen when she pressed any button. In effect, she'd learn nothing about the causation. But children do learn about causal relationships from playing with toys – for example, bouncing and rolling balls, or building towers of bricks and knocking them down – and this is surely related to the observed regularity in these phenomena.

Young Children

Learning a language depends on regularity. Imagine trying to teach a young child the meaning of the word "blue" if each time the objects pointed to were of different colours. Consider what would happen if, when teaching them how to add simple numbers, we gave them different answers each time. Imagine, too, that when teaching a child a song, we varied the melody each time it was played.

We show children how to mix colours to produce a different one. Blue and yellow mixed together make green. But what would it be like if the addition of blue to yellow produced green only 10% of the time, various other colours being observed in the remaining 90% of cases? They would learn nothing about the results of mixing colours. Without regularity, children wouldn't be able to learn about causation.

Older children

In school, science is taught with experiments. Children learn that an acid neutralises an alkali. The experiment is simple: a flask contains a solution of sodium hydroxide and an indicator; when sufficient hydrochloric acid has been added, all of the alkali is neutralised and the indicator changes colour. This outcome always occurs. It never fails. If each child in the classroom repeats the experiment, they will all obtain the same result. This is how they learn. But what if the reaction was only observed in a few cases?

Such demonstrations aren't confined to physics, chemistry and biology lessons. Learning to play the violin, they experience directly the connection between varying the length of the string and alterations in the pitch of the note – regular, predictable causal relationships. Playing snooker, they see at first hand the consistent effects of various different types of collision between the balls and how the outcome depends on the angle of impact and the spin put on the cue ball.

Science, music and sport are just a few of countless activities that develop young people's concept of causation. By the time they leave school, they're equipped with a range of words and phrases by which to express causal concepts. They are fully fledged causal language users.

Causal language in everyday life

When we use causal language in everyday discourse, it's not always obvious from the words and expressions that we are talking about causation. But, if we look closely at what we actually say, we see the underlying concepts of cause and effect relationships. Causal language is complicated and amongst the many ways in which the concept may be expressed, the use of words such as "cause" and "effect" is uncommon. Consider the following examples of causal language:

- We see the child struggling and explain, "You have to squeeze the tube. Like this. Squeezing the tube makes the toothpaste come out. See? Now, you have a go."
- The mechanic listened to the story and then, after a quick look at the car, argued his case. "The lights work… and so do the indicators and the wipers… it's not the battery. And there's no noise when the ignition key's turned… It must be the starter motor. It's jammed."
- The doctor didn't believe the patient. "But you must have been abroad sometime. You've got malaria."
- "If you hadn't switched the heating off before we went away, the pipes wouldn't have frozen."

- After half-an-hour of trying unsuccessfully, the child became irritated. But his father knew what was wrong. "Yes, it will work. But you must focus the sunlight onto the paper. Like this... slowly move the magnifying glass away until you can see the rays concentrated. See? Now you do it. Hold it still... Look, it's starting to smoulder. I told you it always works."

In these examples, unfamiliar or complicated words are absent. The ideas of necessary and sufficient causes are not formerly expressed but they are present all the same. The example of the frozen pipes is nothing but a straightforward counterfactual conditional.

There's never any mention of regularity but it's there in each case. If we were asked, we would agree that squeezing the tube always produces toothpaste. But this doesn't mean that we can't imagine circumstances in which this would not occur. We could describe such conditions – a flaw in the manufacture of the tube or the presence of a foreign object in the nozzle preventing the toothpaste from escaping. Under normal conditions, though, we would say that squeezing the tube is a sufficient cause. And we would surely all agree that water never freezes above a certain temperature. For the most part, regularity is left unsaid. But it may be brought out by simple questions that will show clearly that it lies behind our causal thinking and language.

It's also noticeable that instances of causation in everyday language often include the element of showing – in other words, demonstrating the effect. Much of our causal language involves – implicitly or explicitly – the idea of action and intervention. When we doubt what someone else asserts, we ask for evidence; when someone else doubts what we say, we offer evidence. The possibility of showing the effect is inseparable from the way in which we speak about causation. And, of course, showing or demonstrating a causal relationship depends on regularity.

There's a further aspect to causation that shouldn't be neglected. When we look at language, we see that many of the situations in which we use causal concepts relate to science. This isn't always obvious; sometimes the link is tenuous but, if we look, we can still find it.

The absence of technical terms may be thought of as threatening the accurate communication of causal ideas. But this isn't the case. We're so accustomed to causal discourse that we have no difficulty in understanding the often elliptical – and even cryptic – use of causal language. Sometimes, of course, the utterances may at first be misunderstood. But this doesn't matter; misunderstandings are easily cleared by up enquiries and clarification. That's the way our language works in general and it's no different in the context of causation.

- Although the family had raised questions about the man's treatment in police custody, the coroner decided that the cause of death was a heart attack.
- The enquiry into the Challenger disaster concluded that the cause was the failure of the O-rings.

These last two examples are used in a formal setting where experts are involved in the judgment. This is reflected in the use of the word "cause" which is much less commonly encountered in everyday conversation. Nevertheless, in each case, we can understand what is involved. We know that heart attacks result in death and we know that the post mortem is able to prove conclusively that it occurred. We know, too, that the O-rings were supposed to serve a particular function and that their properties were altered by the low temperatures on the morning of the launch. The heart attack and the faulty O-rings were each responsible for the outcome.

Regularity is everywhere around us, so much so that we fail to see it – no wonder so many people find it easy to reject Hume. But our actions and speech reveal its presence in innumerable instances of causation in the course of our lives. At breakfast, we boil the kettle and make toast. At the table, we pick up the mobile and type out a text message, scrolling up and down to check its accuracy before selecting the appropriate phone number and pressing the send button. Before leaving, we set the alarm and lock the front door. Outside, we scrape the ice of the windscreen and de-mist the rear window before switching on the ignition and accelerating down the road. We indicate right and then turn the steering wheel to overtake. We adjust the heating and change the radio station. In the distance, we see a police car and brake to keep within the speed limit... We could continue in the same vein, commenting on our actions throughout the routine of our daily lives and showing how they reflect our knowledge of cause and effect relationships. The world around us is teeming with regularity.

The features of causation identified earlier – namely, regularity and intervention – are easily recognised in what we say and what we do. Our use of language says all that needs to be said about the subject. We have sufficient knowledge about causation to manipulate the world around us.

Conclusions

Hume's theory of causation has stood the test of time. It's survived, albeit somewhat battered and bruised, for more than 250 years. There's been no shortage of criticism, especially in recent times, but opponents of the regularity theory have little to offer in terms of a better account. The alternatives are either defective or, for the most part, irrelevant.

If we're to respond to the world around us, if we're to manipulate our surroundings to our advantage, then causation is fundamental. Hume fully recognises its importance. It follows, therefore, that whatever the mechanism for identifying a cause and effect relationship, it must be reliable and trustworthy.

Hume locates the grounds for causal inference in our psychological make-up, in our nature. It's primarily an automatic response to certain features in our experience. We simply have a disposition to interpret a particular pattern of observations – namely, the regular occurrence of events of type A followed by events of type B – in terms of causation. Whether this disposition came about by an act of God or Nature – using, perhaps, evolutionary processes – is immaterial. What matters is that this is just what we do. What also matters is that it works. When we successfully identify a causal relationship on the basis of strict regularity, it is reliable and supports accurate predictions.

But the regularity theory by itself isn't enough. We require something more than mere observation. Causation is about practical matters. It's about knowing what will happen when we perform a particular action. And the best way to discover this is by performing the action. Intervention is the crucial contact with the natural world. If all we have is passive observation, then we are divorced from the reality of the events. But manipulating the conditions and observing the outcome tests our ideas of a causal relationship. It confirms or refutes our hypotheses.

The scientific experiment is the archetypal case of causation. It displays regularity in terms of the outcome both in the presence and in the absence of the cause. It involves the deliberate manipulation of the conditions. It also supports universal causal generalisations and permits accurate prediction. The scientific method is a sophisticated and formal approach to the investigation of causal phenomena. But, in terms of its basic principles, it is little different from what we do in our everyday lives.

Hume's regularity theory, supplemented by intervention, offers an approach to the identification of causal relationships which is entirely in keeping with that of science and everyday life.

References

1. Hume D. *A Treatise of Human Nature (1739).* Penguin Books Ltd, Middlesex, England. 1969.
2. Hume D. *An Enquiry into Human Understanding (1748).* Oxford University Press. Oxford, England. 1975.
3. *Ibid.* Hume D. *Treatise.* Page 124.
4. *Ibid.* Hume D. *Enquiry.* Pages 73-74.
5. Ducasse CJ. On the nature and the observability of the causal relation. Journal of Philosophy 1026;23;57-68.
6. Anscombe GEM. Causality and determination. Cambridge University Press, 1971.
7. Harre R, Madden EH. Causal Powers: A theory of natural necessity. Oxford, England. Blackwell, 1975.
8. *Ibid.* Hume D. *Treatise.* Pages 154-5.
9. *Ibid.* Hume D. *Treatise.* Page 135.
10. *Ibid.* Hume D. *Treatise.* Page 138.
11. *Ibid.* Hume D. *Treatise.* Page 198.
12. *Ibid.* Hume D. *Treatise.* Page 137.
13. *Ibid.* Hume D. *Enquiry.* Pages 29-30.
14. *Ibid.* Hume D. *Treatise.* Page 205-6.
15. Scriven M. Defects of the necessary condition analysis of causation. In: Philosophical Analysis and History. Ed W Dray. Harper Collins, 1966.
16. Davidson D. Causal relations. Journal of Philosophy 1967;64;691-703.
17. Mackie JL. The Cement of the Universe. Oxford University Press. Oxford, 1974.
18. Locke J. *An Essay Concerning Human Understanding (1690).* Edited by JW Yolton. Guernsey Press Co. Ltd. 1976. Book II; Chapter XXVI; Page 155.
19. *Ibid.* Hume D. *Treatise.* Pages 206-7.
20. *Ibid.* Hume D. *Treatise.* Pages 213-4.
21. *Ibid.* Hume D. *Enquiry.* Pages 37-8.
22. *Ibid.* Hume D. *Treatise.* Page 140.
23. *Ibid.* Hume D. *Enquiry.* Page 49.

24. *Ibid.* Hume D. *Treatise.* Page 215.
25. *Ibid.* Hume D. *Enquiry.* Page 43.
26. *Ibid.* Hume D. *Treatise.* Pages 154-5.
27. Bennet J. *Locke, Berkeley, Hume: Central Themes.* Oxford University Press. Oxford, 1971.
28. *Ibid.* Hume D. *Enquiry.* Pages 44-5.
29. *Ibid.* Hume D. *Enquiry.* Pages 54-5.
30. Spelke ES, Philips A, Woodward AL. Infants knowledge of object motion and human action. In: Sperber D, Premack D, Premack AJ (Eds). Causal Cognition. Oxford University Press. Oxford, 1995, pp 44-78.
31. Baillargeon R, Kotovsky L, Neeham A. The acquisition of physical knowledge in infancy. In: Sperber D, Premack D, Premack AJ (Eds). Causal Cognition. Oxford University Press. Oxford, 1995, pp 79-116.
32. Schulz LE, Gopnik A. Causal learning across domains. Developmental Psychology 2004;40;162-76.
33. White PA. Ideas about causation in philosophy and psychology. Psychological Bulletin 1990;108;3-18.
34. Glymour C. Learning causes: psychological explanations of causal explanation. Minds and Machines 1998;8;39-60.
35. Michotte AE. The Perception of Causality. Methuen & Co Ltd, London, 1963. Ed CA Mace. Originally published as La Perception de la Causalite. 1946.
36. *Ibid.* Hume D. *Treatise.* Page 220.
37. *Ibid.* Hume D. *Enquiry.* Pages 76-7.
38. Lewis D. Causation. Journal of Philosophy 1973;70;556-67.
39. Kim J. Causes and Counterfactuals. Journal of Philosophy 1973;70;570-2.
40. Horwich P. Lewis' programme. In: Asymmetries in Time: Problems in the Philosophy of Science. Massachusetts Institute of Technology Press. 1987. Pages 167-76.
41. Mackie JL. Counterfactuals and causal laws. In: Analytic Philosophy. Ed RJ Butler. Pages 66-80.
42. *Ibid.* Hume D. *Treatise.* Page 209.

43. Salmon WC. Causality: Production and Propagation. In: Proceedings of the 1980 Biennial Meeting of the Philosophy of Science Association. Vol 2; pages 49-69.
44. *Ibid.* Hume D. *Enquiry*. Pages 69-70.
45. *Ibid.* Hume D. *Enquiry*. Page 31.
46. *Ibid.* Hume D. *Enquiry*. Pages 29-30.
47. *Ibid.* Hume D. *Enquiry*. Pages 57-59.
48. *Ibid.* Hume D. *Enquiry*. Pages 69-70.
49. *Ibid.* Hume D. *Treatise*. Page 225.
50. von Wright GH. *Causality and Determinism*. New York: Columbia University Press, 1974.

XI

Imperfect Causal Inference

The basic tenet of medical research involving statistical studies is that, provided the other conditions for internal validity are established, a statistically significant difference in outcome between the groups indicates the presence of a causal relationship. No limit is set on the size of the difference – as long as it achieves statistical significance, causal inference is justified. This is all taken very much as a matter of course. Yet, it's far from obvious that this approach justifies causal inference. It's certainly not, for example, self-evidently the case.

Causal inferences based on statistical data are ultimately grounded in the probabilistic theory of causation. Much has been written about this over the past fifty years or more and it's gained widespread acceptance in many different fields of research. Given the extent of its influence, it might be expected that the probabilistic theory of causation is without significant problems. Nothing could be further from the truth.

Probabilistic Causation

The basic idea

The fundamental feature of the probabilistic theory of causation is that a cause increases the probability of its effect. This is expressed in terms of conditional probabilities.

C is the cause of E if P[E/C] > P[E/non-C]

A causal relationship between the event C and another event E may be inferred when the probability of E in the presence of C is greater than the probability E in the absence of C.

By itself, however, this isn't enough for the establishment of causation. For example, it fails to address the issue of the asymmetry between a cause and its effect and it's inadequate to deal with the problem of spurious causal relationships. In addition, situations are described where a cause may be observed not to increase the probability of its effect.

The literature relating to probabilistic causation comprises, for the most part, accounts of the conditions for legitimate causal inference together with various counter-examples used to argue that these conditions fail in their purpose. Versions of probabilistic causation first appeared in the mid-20th century. The notable accounts by Reichenbach,[1] Good[2] and Suppes[3] all subscribe to the principle that a cause raises the probability of its effect and address the problems of asymmetry and spurious causes. However, elsewhere they differ. For example, while Reichenbach's aim is to establish a theory of causation without presupposing temporal order, Suppes accepts without question that a cause precedes its effect. Following Reichenbach's original account, these theories consist of a set of conditions presented in terms of equations and relationships of inequality made up of conditional probabilities that are designed to address the problems facing the probability theory of causation.

The problem of asymmetry

One of the difficulties of probabilistic causation is that its definition in terms of a cause raising the probability of its effect doesn't have the necessary asymmetry for a causal relationship.

In normal circumstances, we accept that if C causes E, then E doesn't cause C – the relationship is asymmetrical. But, according to the probabilistic account, if a cause raises the probability of its effect, then it follows that the effect raises the probability of the cause. Thus, the normal asymmetrical relationship between cause and effect is missing and, consequently, a cause can't be distinguished from its effect.

Some accounts – in particular, those that accept that a cause is temporally prior to its effect – offer a way out of this problem. Alternatively, accepting the role of intervention in the clarification of causal relationships provides a solution to the problem of asymmetry. However, this approach, as we've already seen, doesn't find favour with many philosophers.

The problem of spurious causes

Reichenbach introduces the idea of "screening-off" in an attempt to deal with spurious causal relationships.[1] Consider a frequently used example of a spurious cause: from the observation that a fall in the barometer reading is followed shortly afterwards by a storm, it's inferred that the first event causes the second; but the fall in the barometer reading is screened off from the storm by changes in the atmospheric conditions which precede both the storm and the fall in barometer readings.

It's certainly true that the finding that one event raises the probability of another doesn't entail that a causal relationship is present. They may both may the product of a common cause. As Suppes observes, we have to exclude this possibility.

> "... one event is the cause of another if the appearance of the first event is followed with a high probability by the appearance of the second, and there is no third event that we can use to factor out the probability relationship between the first and second events." [3]

Once again, the problem is believed to be solved by a set of conditional probabilities which is applied in order to determine whether or not the causal relationship is spurious.

Does a cause always increase the probability of its effect?

There is, however, another aspect of this theory which has stimulated much discussion and this concerns the question of whether a cause always raises the probability of its effect.

Consider, for instance, the case of oral contraceptives. It's believed, on the basis of epidemiological studies, that contraceptives are one of the causes of thrombo-embolic disease. But pregnancy, too, is a recognised risk factor for this condition. If pregnancy increases the risk more than oral contraceptives, then, given that these drugs prevent pregnancy, they will reduce the overall risk of thrombo-embolic disease. Hence, we have an instance where a cause lowers the probability of its effect. Although counter-arguments have been made, many believe that this sort of example militates against the strict definition of a cause as being something that increases the probability of its effect.[4]

General criticisms

While much has been written about probabilistic causation, its content may easily be considered trivial. There seems to be a good deal of cleverness and no small amount of playing games – the development of increasingly complex theories provoking ever more obscure counter-examples which, in turn, prompt equally intricate defences. Most people who have approached the subject will rapidly become acquainted with Rosen's example of the golfer who slices his shot only to see the ball ricochet off the branch of a tree and land in the hole for a birdie – proof, it's claimed, that Reichenbach's definition of screening-off is flawed.

Other entertaining examples are drawn from activities such as gambling in the casino and playing pool.[4]

What's clear is that the probabilistic theory of causation is found wanting and is not universally accepted.[4] The problems of asymmetry and spurious causation haven't been resolved, while instances of causes lowering the probability of their effects continue to present a challenge. However, the most fundamental question remains, namely, whether a small but statistically significant difference legitimises causal inference in the context of statistics-based research.

Hume and Probabilistic Causation

When it comes to the more marginal regions of causation – most notably, in statistics-based research – Hume has a significant contribution to make. His discussion of the subject centres on what he refers to as a "contrariety" of observations, in other words, the inconsistent relationship between a supposed cause and its effect.

> "Twou'd be happy for men in the conduct of their lives and actions, were the same objects always conjoin'd together, and we had nothing to fear but the mistakes of our own judgment, without having any reason to apprehend the uncertainty of nature. But as 'tis frequently found, that one observation is contrary to another, and that causes and effects follow not in the same order, of which we have had experience, we are oblig'd to vary our reasoning on account of this uncertainty, and take into consideration the contrariety of events." [5]

The confidence that we normally have in the inferring the presence of a cause and effect relationship from observations showing strict regularity is now threatened. Our beliefs about the matter are, in his view,[6,7] "imperfect" and "hesitating" but, nevertheless, we continue to draw causal inferences based on the expectation that the future will resemble this irregular past.

> "...when in considering past experiments we find them of a contrary nature, this determination, tho' full and perfect in itself, presents us with no steady object, but offers us a number of disagreeing images in a certain order and proportion... Any of these past events may happen again; and we judge, that when they do happen, they will be mix'd in the same proportion as in the past." [8]

Here we see the nascent idea of statistical causation: the tendency that we have to project previously irregular experience of causal relationships into the future. We act as though causation will be present in equal proportions in the future to those in the past. But why should we believe this?

Where regularity exists, we have a homogeneous class of objects or events with respect to the outcome. But this isn't the case when we're dealing with matters of probability. Here, we draw inferences from a heterogeneous class. In these circumstances, we have no means of distinguishing the different subgroups within the class – if we could do so, then we would be in a position to subdivide the class into homogeneous groups and study these separately. Consequently, we can't know that the proportions of the different objects or events in the past will be the same in the future.

In the following quotation, Hume says all that's needed to be said about probabilistic causation.

> "... all kinds of reasoning from causes or effects are founded on two particulars, viz. the constant conjunction of any two objects in all past experience, and the resemblance of a present object to any one of them... If you weaken either the union or the resemblance, you weaken the principle of transition, and of consequence that belief, which arises from it... Without some degree of resemblance,

> as well as union, 'tis impossible there can be any reasoning; but as this resemblance admits of many different degrees, the reasoning becomes proportionately more or less firm and certain." [9]

Causal inference depends on regularity and resemblance. When both are present to the greatest degree, causal inference is reliable. But when the objects or events that constitute a causal relationship lose their close resemblance to one another, the reliability of the inference lessens. What Hume is describing is a spectrum of circumstances ranging from perfect resemblance and regularity at one end, to an absence of resemblance and regularity at the other. At some point along this spectrum, the notion of causation is lost.

In Search of Grounds for Probabilistic Causation

Is the idea that the demonstration of a small, statistically significant difference permits causal inference related to the other theories of causation or is it something entirely different? Given the problems with probabilistic causation, this question has particular relevance.

By way of attempting to locate the grounds for probabilistic causation within existing theories, consider a hypothetical RCT designed to assess the efficacy of a new drug in reducing mortality from a common disease in 30,000 patients. Of those given the drug, 4% died during five years of follow-up compared with 5% of those allocated to placebo. The absolute reduction in mortality of 1% was statistically significant. In these circumstances, the small difference in outcome is said to be caused by the treatment. But is the justification for this inference to be found in one of the other theories of causation discussed in the previous chapter?

Direct perception of causation

The theory that we directly perceive causation in the single instance cannot possibly apply to RCTs. In the above example, the 1% of patients who are believed to have benefited from the drug is lost in the 96% of the active treatment group who survived throughout the study. No single individual in whom the outcome was prevented could ever be identified. Hence, even if we were to accept the theory of causation based on the single case, it couldn't provide grounds for probabilistic causation.

Necessary and sufficient causes

Given the results from both the placebo and active treatment groups, it's clear that the drug is neither sufficient nor necessary for survival in the patients studied. Ninety-five percent of those receiving placebo survived; hence, the drug isn't necessary. Four percent of patients receiving active treatment died; hence the drug isn't sufficient to ensure survival.

Necessary and sufficient conditions have no place in statistical studies and can't be used to support probabilitic causation.

Counterfactual analysis

As noted in the previous chapter, the counterfactual analysis is applied to single instances of causation. In the case of the RCT above, a counterfactual statement would assert that, for a particular individual, if he hadn't taken the drug, then he would have died. But this claim can't be made. Firstly, it would require that all patients without treatment would die which is clearly not the case. And, secondly, there would be no possible way of identifying any member of the active treatment group in whom this claim would be true.

It may be thought that expressing the consequent of the counterfactual conditional in terms of a probabilistic statement would solve the first of these problems. But this would still require a generalisation as grounds for the consequent of the counterfactual statement. In other words, it entails reference to causation established by non-counterfactual means. It's difficult, therefore, to understand how probabilistic causation could be grounded on the counterfactual approach.

Probabilistic causation in relation to the regularity theory

What remains is the regularity theory. Hume, as we've seen, accommodates probabilistic causation within a spectrum of varying regularity. But there's nothing in his writings to suggest that he would accept the type of causation involved in large-scale statistical studies. When discussing the subject, he implies that the situations under consideration contain regularity with only a minority of contrary instances. This is very different from modern-day statistical causation. How, then, could the regularity theory provide a basis for probabilistic causation?

Contrived regularity

In all large-scale RCTs, most of the participants are irrelevant to the determination of the effect. The majority don't develop the outcome when left untreated and, consequently, the effect of the drug is tested on a small subgroup of those recruited to the study. It's clear that we do think in terms of these subgroups. Both in the trial protocol beforehand and the paper published afterwards, reference is made to the proportion of patients developing the outcome in the placebo and active treatment groups. These figures define subgroups.

There's a temptation to believe that we can infer causation from these subgroups in isolation from the main body of the study participants. Take the patients who develop the outcome – 5% with placebo, 4% with active treatment. It's easy to imagine that there's strict regularity in terms of the outcome in the subgroups. As for the difference in outcome of 1%, this defines the subgroup who benefit from treatment and it would appear that there is strict regularity with respect to the presence of the active drug and the outcome in this subgroup. This, though, is a faulty analysis. These subgroups are defined by the presence of the outcome. But, when we're investigating causation, the reference class must be defined by exposure to the cause and not by the occurrence of the effect. By defining the reference class in terms of the effect, the observed regularity is purely contrived.

For the purpose of causal analysis, the groups formed by randomisation can't be divided into subgroups defined by the occurrence of the outcome. If there are features which would allow recognition of the participants who would develop the outcome, then the study should be restricted to these patients alone. If not, any attempt to use the outcome in order to define subgroups precludes causal analysis.

We have to restrict the analysis of causal relationships to the whole groups formed by randomisation. But, from this, it follows that there's no regularity – certainly no regularity in the conventional sense of the word – in large-scale RCTs. The notion of regularity relates to the correlation between the presence of the cause and the presence of the effect or between the absence of the cause and the absence of its effect. Strict regularity requires a one-to-one correlation. But even lesser degrees of regularity are missing in statistic causation.

Ignoring the true regularity

Paradoxically, if we examine the entire results of a large RCT, what strikes us immediately is that most patients remain free from the outcome. In the above example, 95% of patients survived without active treatment. Surely, if we are to speak of regularity, then it's to be located in this observation. It allows us to predict, with reasonable accuracy, that the outcome in any individual patient will be favourable regardless of treatment. This is a useful finding although it has nothing to do with identifying causal relationships.

Locating Statistics-Based Research in Hume's spectrum

As already noted, Hume's writings suggest a spectrum of cases from that of perfect regularity at one end to an absence of regularity at the other. This idea of a range of possible situations is observed as we pass from experiments in the physical sciences to statistics-based studies in medicine.

Hume's Spectrum

	Strict regularity	One-sided heterogeneity		Two-sided heterogeneity
Cause absent	0%	>0%	0%	>0%
Cause present	100%	100%	<100%	<100%
	Effect occurs			

From cases of strict regularity, we can infer the present of causation, make universal generalisations and show the causal relationship in individual instances. In addition, external validity presents no problem.

One-sided heterogeneity allows some of these conclusions, depending on which side the irregularity occurs. If all our experiences – including the results of other experiments – show that the effect never occurs in absence of the cause, then we may infer causation in those cases where the effect occurs in the presence of the cause. This isn't the case when the irregularity resides in the controls because we could not be certain that the effect would not have occurred in the absence of the cause.

When two-sided heterogeneity is present, the conclusions are uncertain and this uncertainty worsens as the heterogeneity increases. For example, if the effect occurs in the absence of the cause in only 5% whilst it is present in 95% of instances where the cause is present, then it would seem reasonable to assume a causal relationship provided other aspects of internal validity are satisfied. This would be acceptable in the context of medical research; it would certainly have practical value. As the heterogeneity increases further, our tendency to infer causation diminishes. In a situation where the outcome occurs in 60% with the cause and 40% without it, we would be reluctant to infer a causal relationship unless we could be very sure that the only difference between the groups was that of the causal factor. But once we enter the realms of extreme heterogeneity – as, for example, in the above RCT – none of the conclusions that follow from strict regularity apply and there's little to support the presence of a causal relationship.

As we move further and further away from regularity and resemblance – that is, in the direction of statistics-base research with its emphasis on large studies with small treatment differences – the validity of causal inference decreases to the point where it is non-existent.

The Loss of Contact with Causal Events

It seems, therefore, that probabilistic causation isn't grounded in any other recognised theory and, as such, must stand alone. This is an unpalatable conclusion. Even if we ignore the problems associated with internal and external validity, the absence of any independent means of testing the methodology is sufficient to raise serious questions about its validity. Perhaps, if it had delivered striking advances in medicine over many years, we might feel more comfortable about accepting an unsupported theory. But there's no history of endless successes, only exaggerated claims based on trivial treatment effects that can't be confirmed. In short, if we don't accept the fundamental idea that a cause is something that raises the probability of its effect, then there's little else outside of the probabilistic theory of causation that can convince us.

However, the inference from a small, statistically significant difference to the presence of a causal relationship isn't self-evidently true. It's not a truth based on logic or meaning. There are many reasons for being sceptical about causal inference in this context, as discussed in the present chapter. And there is a further obstacle.

Causation concerns events in the natural world. It's an empirical matter and knowledge of causal relationships is grounded in experience. For a theory of causation to be sound, it must be closely tied to the happenings in the world around us. But does this condition apply to statistics-based research?

Projecting the method indefinitely

Clearly, many people believe in probabilistic causation. Some of these accept it unthinkingly at face value, while others are indoctrinated by long exposure to an environment in which it's considered established practice. But there's little doubt that, to many, the notion that a cause is something that raises the probability of its effect appears to be unproblematic.

The origin of the problem lies in our tendency to move along Hume's spectrum without any thought for the consequences. We accept that strict regularity isn't always present and, at the same time, we recognise that minor deviations from this situation don't prevent us drawing useful causal inferences. In the biological sciences, for example, if we observe that the effect occurs in 5% of cases without the cause and in 95% with the cause, we have identified a valuable causal relationship. We don't require statistics – we can judge the presence of causation ourselves. The trouble starts as the proportions become closer together and as the differences in outcome become smaller. Blinkered by statistics, we forget everything else that's involved in causation and focus instead on significance tests and hypothesis tests. If we're not concerned about anything else, we can increase the size of a study indefinitely in order to ensure that very small differences reach statistical significance and, hence, that a causal relationship is established.

The mistake is to believe that a causal relationship may be inferred solely on the basis of a statistically significant difference. This is the decisive move that severs the tie between causation and events in the natural world.

The missing experience

Identifying causation involves observing instances of the cause followed by the effect and instances of the absence of the effect when the cause doesn't occur. These links are what we expect of causation. They are also what constitute a scientific experiment. But they are missing from statistical causation. For example, as has been repeatedly emphasized, we can never identify any instance of treatment success in statistics-based research although we are able to identify individuals in whom treatment has failed.

The dislocation between experience and causal inference may be further appreciated by considering our response to the data the end of the trial. If we are shown the complete list of individual results, we can calculate the proportions of those who developed the outcome in each group and find the difference. But we can go no further. We can't draw any causal inference without the statistical analysis. This shows how judgments about causal relationships in large-scale RCTs are not grounded in our experience of events in the natural world. Instead, they are the product of statisticians who have never encountered a single patient in the study, who may know next to nothing about the disease or the treatment, but who have been given the bare numbers and asked to deliver their verdict.

Alternatively, we might look at the data from a large-scale RCT in a different way. Consider viewing the results in pairs. This has nothing to do with paired statistical analysis but is merely a way of inspecting the data visually. Each pair contains the outcome for one patient in the placebo group and one receiving the active drug. If the outcome is present, then that member of the pair is marked Y; if it is absent, it is marked N. The thousands of pairs are printed and inspected. In the above RCT showing mortality of 5% in the placebo group reduced to 4% with the active drug, most pairs will be NN; a small percentage will be NY or YN; very few will be YY. On looking at this display of the data, there would be nothing to convince us of the presence of any causal relationship between the active drug and the outcome. Indeed, if we didn't know in advance, we couldn't tell with any confidence which group was which. Now, consider a similar display of data from a physics or chemistry experiment. Every single pair would be NY, showing individual instances of cause and effect relationship. This is a stark reminder of the difference in causal inference between situations were there is strict regularity and resemblance, and those where the study sample is heterogeneous and without any discernible regularity.

That statistics-based research is divorced from the individual events is of the utmost importance. Causation is precisely about these events and, when they are ignored, the inferences that we draw are no longer secure.

Conclusions

From its inception, the probabilistic theory of causation has faced obstacles. The concept of probability-raising is, by itself, unable to provide the necessary asymmetry between cause and effect, it's unable to exclude spurious causation, and faces a challenge from cases where a cause fails to increase the probability of its effect. These problems have not yet been resolved although it should be acknowledged that, in the context of RCTs, they're of less importance.

This, though, is far from the end of the difficulties. As we've seen, it isn't possible to ground the probabilistic account in terms of any of the other recognised theories of causation. It must, therefore, be judged in its own right.

Does statistics-based research deliver success? Has the methodology produced important scientific advances? There is little evidence that either observational studies or large-scale RCTs have done so. In fact, the nature of these studies is such that the treatment effects are necessarily very small. Can we have confidence in the results of this type of research? Given the absence of any method to confirm or refute the results of a particular study, we can't know that they are valid. More importantly, there's no independent way of testing the statistical method of research in general.

How does statistics-based research fit in with our everyday understanding of causation? Compared with our ordinary ideas of causation or those involved in most of scientific research, the probabilistic approach is seen to be very different. Again, this is of importance. We understand and trust the causal inferences that we make; we have good reason to do so. For the most part, our causal judgements are reliable and allow us to predict future outcomes. If probabilistic causation showed similarities with our everyday and scientific approach to causation, then we might have more faith in it. But they have little in common.

The basic tenet of statistical causation is that, in the context of observational studies or large-scale RCTs, the finding of a small but statistically significant difference is sufficient to draw a causal inference. The advocates of statistics-based research accept this without question. In so doing, they forget how much more is involved. Causation is tied to individual events in the natural world. But statistical research has slipped its mooring and floats free, unfettered by the constraints normally imposed on causal judgments. It bears little resemblance to causation as we know it in everyday life or in the experiments of science. It's of the utmost importance that this distinction is recognised. If some people wish to use the term causation in relation to the conclusions of statistics-based research, there's nothing to stop them. But they mean something entirely different from that of our normal understanding of this concept.

Almost 300 years ago, Hume recognised the problems confronting causal inference when observations are inconsistent. As regularity and resemblance are lost, there is a corresponding weakening of causal inference. If we go to the extreme end of the spectrum, we find ourselves in the territory inhabited by large-scale statistical studies. In this place, legitimate causal inference is nowhere to be found.

References

1. Reichenbach H. The Direction of Time. Berkeley, California & Los Angeles, 1956.
2. Good IJ. A causal calculus. British Journal for the Philosophy of Science 1961;11;305-18.
3. Suppes P. A probabilistic theory of causality. Amsterdam, 1970.
4. Salmon WC. Probabilistic causality. Pacific Philosophical Quarterly 1980;61; 50-74.
5. Hume D. *A Treatise of Human Nature (1739).* Penguin Books Ltd, Middlesex, England. 1969. Page 182.
6. *Ibid.* Hume D. *Treatise,* Pages 185-6.
7. *Ibid.* Hume D. *Treatise,* Page 183.
8. *Ibid.* Hume D. *Treatise,* Page 184-5.
9. *Ibid.* Hume D. *Treatise,* Page 192-3.

XII

The Final Reckoning

The arguments presented in this text are varied, wide-ranging and complex. It's now time to see whether the case against statistics-based research has been made successfully. If so, this would have implications far beyond the field of medical research.

The Case against Statistics-Based Research

The Validity of Statistics-Based Research

The fundamental feature of statistics-based research is that the demonstration of a small difference in outcome between the study groups is sufficient to permit causal inference.

The Basic Feature of Statistics-Based Research

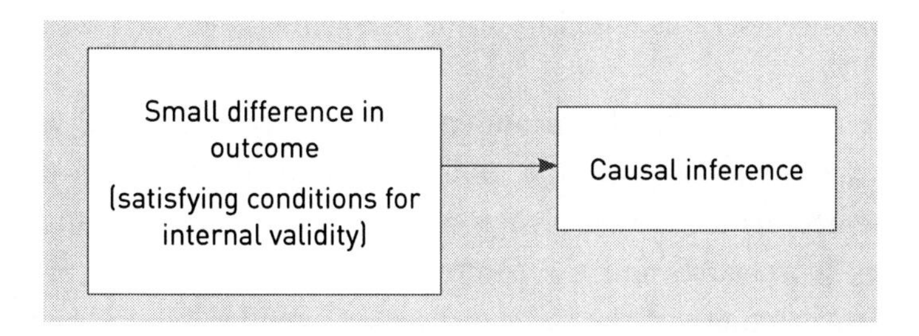

There is an important proviso: all other explanations for the observed difference have to have been ruled out. In other words, the conditions for internal validity – the exclusion of an unequal distribution of relevant factors, bias in the assessment of the outcome and chance – must be satisfied.

The failure of internal validity

Randomisation, allocation concealment, the double-blind technique, intention-to-treat analysis and statistical tests are included in the design of large-scale RCTs with the purpose of ensuring that any observed difference may be attributed to the treatment effect. In practice, however, we can never be confident that other explanations have been excluded.

Faulty mechanisms to achieve internal validity

The mechanisms aimed at ensuring internal validity are far from being foolproof. For instance, randomisation doesn't guarantee that the groups are equally matched in respect of all factors relevant to the outcome. In fact, all of the tools employed to achieve internal validity may malfunction and all are open to abuse. Cases of deliberate interference with randomisation, allocation concealment and blinding have been described, while false reporting of intention-to-treat analysis and the incorrect use of statistical tests are well recognised.

The problem of frequentist statistics

Virtually all of the RCTs and epidemiological studies published in the literature have used frequentist statistics. Yet, amongst statisticians, there has been serious criticism of the frequentist approach for many years.

The confusion and misunderstandings relating to P-values, confidence intervals and the null hypothesis have been widely documented. There are misgivings about the relevance of frequentist statistics to research and the common practice of merging Fisher's significance testing with the Neyman-Pearson hypothesis test. Questions have been raised about the issue of more extreme data as well as the failure to adhere to the assumptions on which statistical tests are based. There is evidence, too, that frequentist methods exaggerate the statistical significance of observed differences. But, perhaps of most concern is that, as time passes, more and more problems are unearthed. We can only guess what else will emerge in future to threaten the conventional approach to statistics.

These doubts about the validity of frequentist methods strike at the heart of the statistics-based research.

Testing statistics-based research

Given the uncertainties about the internal validity of RCTs, it's clear that we need some means of testing the results of individual studies. But, more importantly, a way of independently validating the methodology of statistics-based research in general is required.

Testing the results of individual studies

In the normal course of events, when claims for causation are doubted, evidence is easily produced. In particular, the causal relationship may be demonstrated. Showing that one event produces another is part and parcel of causation. There is nothing mysterious about it. Everything is out in the open.

When considering the results of a large RCT, the single case can never prove that one event causes another. It's impossible to infer from the outcome that it was the consequence of treatment because it's much more likely that it would have occurred without any intervention. Replication isn't an option either, because the conditions of a large-scale RCT can't be recreated. When apparently similar trials yield conflicting results, this is attributed to differences between the studies. But, if one study can't refute the results of another, then neither can it confirm the results of the other. Each large-scale RCT stands alone.

This is welcome news to those individuals intent on research misconduct. While the true extent of fraud in medical research is unknown, recent evidence suggests that it's far more common than hitherto supposed. It's a sobering thought that large-scale RCTs – which offer the greatest financial rewards – aren't open to challenge by independent testing.

Testing the statistical method

Statistical research is designed to be used in situations where there is heterogeneity. The scientific method, on the other hand, relies on homogeneity, on identifying objects and events that, in terms of the outcome, are the same. It's obvious, therefore, that we can't use the scientific method to test the validity of the results of large-scale RCTs. But there's nothing else available. There's no independent way of testing the methodology of statistics-based research.

It would appear, then, that if we are to accept this methodology, we must do so on trust. Yet, as has been repeatedly documented, the actions of many involved in medical research make it difficult to accept their word when it comes to the validity of statistics-based research.

Philosophical objections to statistical causation

The statistical approach is based on the probabilistic theory of causation. The notion of a cause as being something that raises the probability of its effect is recognised to be problematic – particularly with reference to the asymmetry of causal relationships and the presence of spurious causes. However, in the context of RCTs, these problems are of less importance. The crucial issue concerns the grounds for causal inference.

The grounds for causation in statistics-based research

From the widespread acceptance of statistics-based research, it would appear that few people have difficulty with the notion that a small, statistically significance difference in outcome justifies causal inference. But this isn't self-evidently true. It's certainly inconsistent with other theories of causation. Why, then, is it so readily taken at face value?

Perhaps, the answer lies in the perceived resemblance between statistics-based research and science. In many ways, a scientific experiment and a RCT are similar. Both involve deliberate intervention and a control group. And they share a common purpose in the identification of causal relationships. It's easy, therefore, to take the statistical approach as simply a variation of the scientific method. But we should be wary of doing so as the differences between the two are substantial.

Causation in science

Science, as practised for hundreds of years, has been associated with enormous advances in knowledge and delivered numerous technological innovations that have improved our lives. Its success rests on the idea that research should focus on the investigation of homogeneous classes. Using pre-existing knowledge and established theory, objects and events are selected which, in terms of factors relevant to the outcome, are identical. This homogeneity is the source of strict regularity.

At a stroke, the problems associated with statistics-based research melt away. The concepts of internal validity and external validity are redundant. As the reference class is accurately specified and regularity is present, it follows that the validity of the results of scientific experiments may be tested by replication. Given the regularity in outcome in both the presence and the absence of the cause – 100% and 0%, respectively – the difference between the groups is maximal. Thus, there can be no dispute about the value of the findings. Finally, regularity supports universal generalisations and ensures that predictions derived from the data are reliable.

Causal inference in science is consistent with Hume's regularity theory supplemented by intervention. In principle, it's very similar to our everyday notion of how we identify cause and effect relationships.

Causation in Science

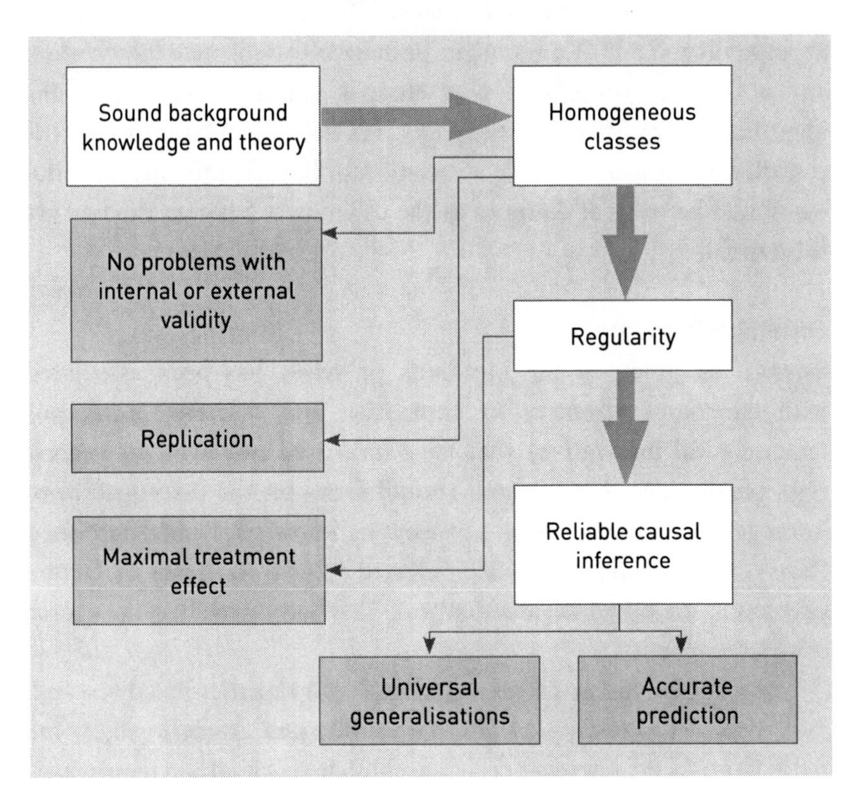

Causation in statistics-based research

In statistics-based research, knowledge of the subject matter is limited and the background theory is weak. The consequence is an inability to identify homogeneous classes. There's no alternative but to accept heterogeneity. But there's a very large price to pay.

All of the problems of internal and external validity stem from the decision to use heterogeneous groups. This also accounts for the inability to confirm the results with replication. More importantly, it leads to a situation in which there can be no independent way of testing the methodology of statistics-based research.

Causation in Statistics-Based Research

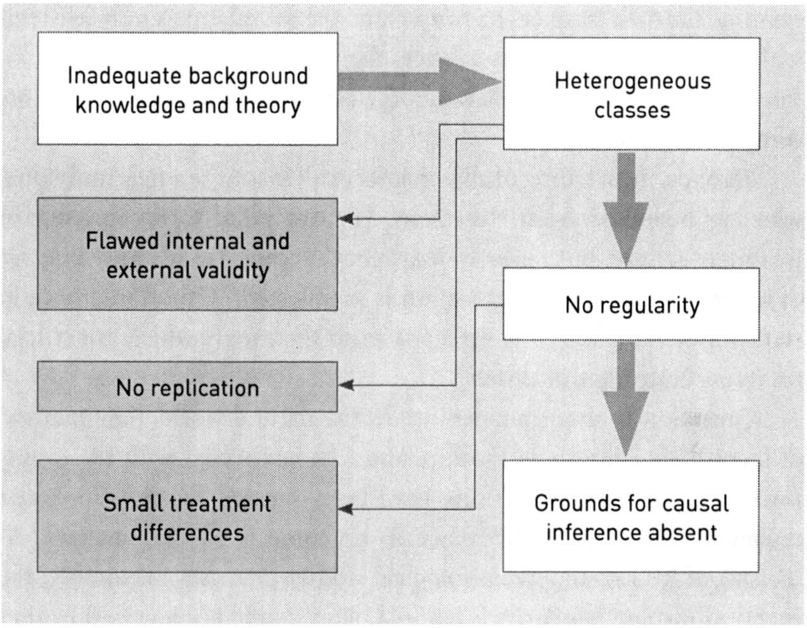

Inadequate background knowledge and theory

Heterogeneous classes

Flawed internal and external validity

No regularity

No replication

Small treatment differences

Grounds for causal inference absent

Without homogeneity, there's no regularity. Instead, everything focuses on the detection of small differences in outcome. As for the other features that are integral to the identification of causal relationships, they are pushed aside. But what do we really know about this small difference?

To begin with, we can never be sure that the difference isn't the result of inequalities between the groups or the product of flaws in frequentist statistics. When we discuss the difference in relation to causal inference, we can't be certain that it's to be attributed to the treatment – indeed, we can't even be certain that it's a genuine difference.

But there's another problem: we don't actually observe a real difference. If we add up all the events in each group and determine the difference, we can't know what it means. We must await the verdict of the statistician. This shows how statistics-based research is divorced from the actual events. Alternatively, if we take a large-scale RCT and examine the data from each group pairs, the causal link is non-existent; with a similar approach in science, the contrast is stark. Once again, this shows the dislocation between the causal judgment and the events comprising causation.

Perhaps, most telling of all is that we can't identify a single individual who has benefited from treatment. We can point to an instance of treatment failure, but never to treatment success. Yet it's only in cases of treatment success that causation is manifested. Causal inference in statistics-based research is detached from the events which are crucial for its accurate identification.

Causation is about happenings in the natural world. Any method of identifying causal relationships must be connected with the events involved. But the connections have been severed in statistics-based research. Nowadays, a difference in outcome is all that matters. As the size of RCTs and epidemiological studies increases inexorably, the ever diminishing regularity is ignored. No thought is given to the other features that contribute to establishing causal relationships.

Hume pointed out that as the conditions move away from strict resemblance and regularity, so the reliability of causal inference decreases. Statistics-based research is located at the opposite end of this spectrum where regularity is nowhere to be seen and causal inference is no longer legitimate.

A Product of Doubtful Value

The claim that statistics-based research has delivered major advances in medicine is a myth. We only have to look at two facets of the large-scale RCT – namely, the external validity of the study and the value of the reported treatment effect – to realise that the product hardly bears the hallmark of genuine success.

The failure of external validity

If we don't know to whom the results apply, then the value of the study is thrown into doubt. This is the problem of external validity that perpetually threatens any generalisation of the results of statistics-based research.

In principle, frequentist statistics apply to classes, not to individuals. Even if a study sample were selected randomly from the wider population of patients, the results only apply to groups. Once identified, an individual is no longer anonymous but, instead, is distinguished from others by characteristics that may be of relevance to the outcome. This is of some concern in the context of medical research which is used in the treatment of individual patients.

In the ideal situation, the study participants would be selected randomly from the whole population of patients with the disease. The results would then apply to future samples selected in a similar manner from the same population. In practice, participants in RCTs are rarely selected randomly. On the contrary they are recruited by processes that inevitably lead to differences between them and the wider population of patients. These differences may be relevant to the outcome and, hence, any generalisation from the results of a RCT to future patients will be flawed.

Ultimately, the failure of external validity is a manifestation of the statistical approach to causation which involves heterogeneous classes. RCTs are performed on samples without any clear idea of the constituents. Furthermore, the absence of selection by randomisation breaks the connection between the sample and the underlying population. Some characteristics may be identified and recorded but a complete description of all the factors that may be related to the outcome isn't possible. In these circumstances, external validity inevitably fails.

The meaning and importance of results to individuals

While researchers eulogise about the importance of their findings, this view isn't shared by patients or, for that matter, by their doctors. When properly informed of the size of the benefits, many patients choose not to have treatment. This is because the small absolute risk reductions make no discernible difference to their lives. In other words, the size of the treatment effect is meaningless.

The obsession with relative risk reductions shows just how sensitive the researchers are to criticism of the size of the absolute risk reductions. They would probably prefer to rid themselves of the charge of misleading patients but the paltry treatment effects necessitate using relative risks. Similarly, focusing on the benefits of treatment in terms of populations creates the impression of a sizeable reduction in outcome but, once again, this is of no relevance to individual patients.

If anything shows the futility of the statistical approach, it is the product delivered by this research. Not only can we never be sure as to which individuals or classes the results apply, but the benefits on offer are next to worthless.

Statistics-Based Research – a Product of Our Times?

In the face of such a damning attack, it has to be wondered how statistics-based research has managed to flourish. No doubt, many people will recoil from these criticisms. They will assume, quite reasonably, that the case in favour of this approach must have been firmly established. After all, academics and researchers the world over accept it, it's taught in all universities, it's a pre-requisite for publication and it's used in a wide range of disciplines. Voices of dissent are few and far between. Indeed, the almost universal adherence to the statistical method may be viewed as a testament to its validity and its worth. But there are other explanations for these observations.

Historical context

RA Fisher's work in statistics and the design of experiments that first appeared in 1925 had an enormous influence on researchers. This was soon followed by developments in the philosophy of science – in particular, the writings of Rudolph Carnap and Karl Popper – that heralded an era of objectivism with an emphasis on logic. By the mid-20th century, the mood of the times favoured the statistical approach to research and many academic spheres duly fell into line. Medicine, in particular, needed no second invitation. Dazzled by promises of solutions to the problems of therapeutic trials and epidemiological studies, researchers eagerly signed up. That these promises were empty, however, has done little to dampen the enthusiasm. A protracted period of indoctrination and endless propaganda have ensured that the failings rarely reach the surface.

Nowadays, the statistical method is the paradigm that governs the thinking of researchers and they're unable to escape its influence. They're under the spell of statistics and the absence of any criticism is only to be expected. But this silence mustn't be interpreted as indicating that all is well. It's certainly not evidence that statistics-based research has delivered notable advances – on the contrary, it's proved to be, for the most part, sterile. Popularity is no guarantee of quality.

The illusion of success

Spin doctors who look after the politicians and media consultants who care for their celebrities are experts in the fields of damage limitation and the creation of success where none actually exists. The advocates of statistics-based research are no different.

Academics and researchers have used all means at their disposal to defend the statistical approach. For example, they increased the size of trials by stealth because of a fear that the sudden introduction of large studies would lead to their rejection. Their lips have been sealed when it comes to the questions raised about frequentist statistics that for so long have remained confined to specialist texts. And they've conducted an endless advertising campaign placing large-scale RCTs at the pinnacle of the hierarchy of evidence while, all the time, they remain silent of the fact that both the validity and the value of a study are inversely proportional to its size. Much that should be out in the open is left unsaid.

When it's in their interest, they have no qualms about using the data selectively, manipulating the results and even drawing false conclusions. Worst of all, they use deceit. We only have to recall the scandal of the colorectal cancer screening programme. The sheer scale of the deceit is hard to believe: millions of healthy individuals cajoled into participating in a screening process with little prospect of benefit. Yet it happened; and it continues to happen.

It would appear that it's better to present data in terms of misleading relative risk reductions than to admit the futility of large-scale RCTs with their trivial absolute risk reductions. It's all about creating the illusion of success.

But data manipulation, trickery and deceit have their downside. Given the doubts about the methodology and the lack of any means of testing its validity, we are left with the option of accepting statistics-based research on the word of its proponents. This is hardly something that we can face with relish.

Preserved by vested interests

But we shouldn't be surprised. So much has been invested by so many different groups over so long that the forces resisting exposure of the flaws in statistics-based research are formidable.

Professors and senior researchers have reputations to protect – reputations built on large-scale RCTs and epidemiological studies. Are we seriously to imagine that they would admit that their work is nothing but a sham? In any case, they have incomes to maintain – not only their salaries and the financial support for their departments but personal monetary gain from close ties with pharmaceutical companies.

No other group has more of a vested interest in the continuation of statistics-based research than the pharmaceutical industry. Their survival depends on products marketed on the basis of the results of RCTs. It's a feature of large-scale trials that they support the use of drugs in substantial sections of the population and, while this involves treating many people without any prospect of benefit, it swells the profits of the drug companies. The power and influence of the pharmaceutical industry make it unlikely that there will be any change in the status quo.

In recent times, the government, too, has instigated programmes – for example, in fields such as the prevention of cardiovascular disease and cancer screening – that are based predominantly on the results of large-scale RCTs. It's hard to believe that these policies will be reversed. Moreover, the health industry is now a major part of the economy – both in terms of the National Health Service and the private pharmaceutical companies. Nothing will be done to damage its interests.

There's simply too much at stake for there to be any realistic expectation of a renunciation of statistics-based research in the near future.

A quick fix

There's an impatience that's endemic in modern society. It manifests itself as a desire for instant gratification and immediate answers. We've come to expect that problems will be solved without delay.

Statistics-based research caters for this need for a quick fix. The availability of large data-bases allows researchers instant access to the raw materials for their next cohort or case-control study. Tens of thousands of participants are no obstacle – the paper is ready for publication within a few months. RCTs take longer than epidemiological studies but still avoid the delays inherent in a more methodical approach involving the identification of homogeneous groups.

From the point of view of those keen to be seen to be doing something – regardless of its value – statistics-based research is a godsend. Forget whether the action is of any benefit, it's all about making an impression that something important has been done. As long as a programme has been put in place, then the politicians are happy; so are the researchers; and so, too, it seems, are the consumers. As for the value, well, that's just something that can be fabricated. What matters is that the boxes are ticked.

Authoritarianism

All data from statistics-based research are open to interpretation. In fact, there's so much latitude that the results may be claimed to support opposing conclusions. This situation is made even worse by the absence of any means of testing either the outcome of an individual study or the methodology in general. The consequences are obvious: what a study shows is determined by the views of those in positions of power and authority. It's the opinion – of the authors and the researchers, of the sponsors, of the editors of journals and referees, and many others – and not the data that determines what is to count as evidence or knowledge.

Bacon and Galileo must be turning in their graves. For more than 300 years, we have accepted their teachings, investigating nature with scientific experiments which are subjected to replication by other researchers. The data – the facts – are objective. The scientific method has delivered previously undreamt of advances. We're able to change the world about us in a predictable manner. Causal relationships are visible, palpable. There's no need for any debate. Then, statistics arrives with data as malleable as warm wax, to be shaped into anything that the powerful and influential want. Results are promoted and advertised. The loudest voices prevail and what they have to say depends on their interests.

In recent times, there's a strong impression of authoritarianism creeping into our lives. We see it in the challenges to the professions – teaching and medicine, to name but two. Trust in individuals is no longer enough. There must be constant surveillance to ensure that they're acting in line with the current orthodoxy. The freedom of professionals to take decisions based on their learning and experience is shunned and strict rules are put in place which, if not adhered to, lead to censure. Statistics-based research fits in well with this new age of authoritarianism. Politicians, NHS managers and others with a vested interest can decide what the data mean and act accordingly. In the case of passive smoking, dubious data were used to enact laws, while millions of healthy individuals have been subjected to the dangers of colorectal cancer screening without evidence of any benefit in overall survival.

But the problem isn't confined to medicine. The use of so-called knowledge where none actually exists is endemic, influencing every aspect of our lives. We're led to believe that the economic forecasts delivered by highly sophisticated computer models produce accurate predictions; but we're all aware of how economists worldwide failed to anticipate the credit crunch. Then we have the meteorologists unable to resist telling the future on the basis of statistical modelling; but, for all the hype, their medium and long-term weather forecasts are no better than those obtained using a crystal ball. And, of course, we have the products of research in the social sciences: miles of shelf space cluttered with textbooks and journals crammed with studies brimful of statistical jargon, formulae and graphs – ideal for the coffee tables of the chattering classes but without any semblance of knowledge.

Our world is infested with nonsense. And the source of much of this is statistics-based research. But the new authoritarians aren't put off by this – in fact, it's just what they want. They don't have to worry about a future study contradicting their position; they know that, whatever the result, it will not be definitive and, hence, will present no real challenge to them. In effect, they are immune to attack by further evidence. Their own opinion, their own interpretation of previous results, will prevail.

Statistics-based research is a crucial weapon in the new authoritarianism. But it isn't science. It's sophistry.

A Final Word

Nowadays, we hear endlessly the mantra that decisions must be evidence-based – as if this were something new. Usually, the evidence referred to is from studies using the statistical approach. It's ironic that, in this era of such deference to evidence, we give so much respect to a methodology that delivers just the opposite. Evidence that's open to interpretation and that can be so readily manipulated is no evidence; evidence that's derived from a flawed method is no evidence; and evidence that can't be tested independently is no evidence.

We shouldn't really expect anything better from statistics-based research. Background knowledge of the subject matter is so limited that it's impossible to identify homogeneous groups and, instead, studies are carried out on collections of individuals that are different from one another in important respects. All of the problems with this type of research stem directly from this decision.

The advocates of the statistical approach argue that they put in place mechanisms to deal with the difficulties arising from heterogeneity but, as we've seen, this is merely tinkering with an intrinsically flawed mechanism. They don't know whether the conditions for internal validity have been satisfied or whether the frequentist approach to statistics is sound. They don't know how to confirm or refute the results of a particular study, or how to test the methodology independently. They don't know to whom the generalisations apply or what the meaning and relevance of the results are to individuals. The source of all the flaws is the acceptance of the notion that anything of value can be reliably extracted from large classes of objects known to be different from one another. And when we delve into the matter, we find that there's no foundation – either in terms of philosophy or common sense – on which to ground statistical causation.

Statistics-based research begins and ends with ignorance. Any claim for knowledge is simply pretence. The process, couched in mathematical symbols and formulae, has the air of exactness and logic, yet its raw materials are imprecise and its methods are dubious while its philosophical basis is elusive. Knowledge is no part of statistics-based research and causal inference is a fiction.

We have been conned. And it's our own fault. We're very gullible. We favour appearance over substance. We submit to advertising and promotion because we're too lazy to ask questions. We're accustomed to being spoon-fed – we don't want to be troubled with having to think about difficult concepts when somebody else will do that for us. Yet we should know better. It's not as though we haven't been warned. We would never have fallen under the spell of statistics if we'd heeded the words of David Hume three centuries ago.

Index

C

D

E

F

L

M

N

O

P

R

S

T

U

V

W

Lightning Source UK Ltd.
Milton Keynes UK
176323UK00001B/31/P